CLARE Hargreaves is currently working in BBC television documentaries. From 1987 until 1992 she was a member of the Diplomatic Staff of *The Daily Telegraph*. In 1990 she won a Journalist Fellowship to Oxford University where she researched and wrote *Snowfields*. Previously she worked for the BBC World Service and Reuters news agency, for whom she was a correspondent in Paris. She has also edited and co-authored a travel book on Chile and Argentina (Bradt Publications 1989). She has travelled extensively in Latin America, and lived and worked in a number of countries including France, Spain, Greece and Peru. She studied at New Hall, Cambridge University, where she took a degree in Spanish and French.

Snowfields

THE WAR ON
COCAINE
IN THE ANDES

★

CLARE HARGREAVES

Snowfields

THE WAR ON COCAINE IN THE ANDES

★

HM

HOLMES & MEIER

Snowfields: The War on Cocaine in the Andes
was first published in 1992.

United States of America
Holmes & Meier Publishers, Inc.,
30 Irving Place,
New York,
NY 10003.

Rest of the World
Zed Books Ltd,
57 Caledonian Road,
London N1 9BU,
United Kingdom.

Copyright © Clare Hargreaves, 1992.

Cover designed by Andrew Corbett.
Cover photograph by Carlos Reyes-Manzo/Andes Press Agency.
Edited and laserset by Selro Publishing Services, Oxford.
Printed and bound in the United Kingdom
by Biddles Ltd, Guildford and King's Lynn.

A catalogue record for this book is
available from the British Library

ISBN 1 85649 077 7 Hb
ISBN 1 85649 078 5 Pb

USA
US CIP information is available
from the Library of Congress

ISBN 0 8419 1327 7 hc
ISBN 0 8419 1328 5 pbk

Contents

Acknowledgements

THIS book was researched and written during a one-year Journalist Fellowship at Queen Elizabeth House, Oxford. I am indebted to Neville Maxwell, the director of the Journalists' Fellowship Programme, and to Max Hastings, the editor of *The Daily Telegraph*, and Nigel Wade, the foreign editor, who generously allowed me a year's leave. Deep thanks are also due to General Gary Prado, the Bolivian ambassador to London, to Jaime Idrovo of UNFDAC in Cochabamba, and to Marcia Paz at the British Embassy in La Paz. Among those who provided invaluable help and insightful comments on the text I should like to thank Laurence Whitehead of Nuffield College, Oxford; Malcolm Deas of St Antony's College, Oxford; James Dunkerley of Queen Mary College, London; Coletta Youngers and John Walsh from the Washington Office on Latin America; Shayne Mitchell; Colin McIntyre; Pilar Domingo; and my father, John Hargreaves. I am grateful to Lucy Hodges and Michael Prest who provided me with a home while I did research in Washington. I should also like to thank my friends and family who gave me support and encouragement. And above all, the scores of Bolivians who were so patient with the visiting *gringa*: without their willingness to share their lives, this book would not be.

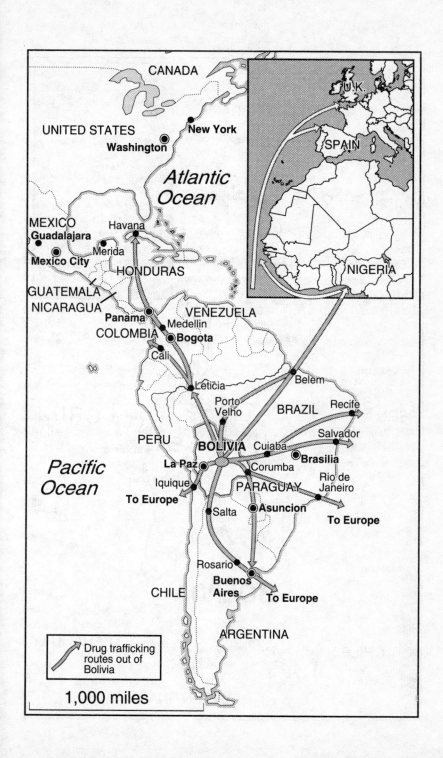

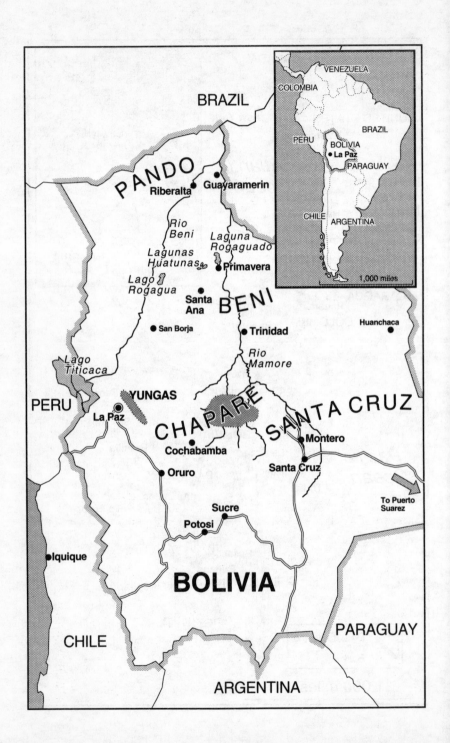

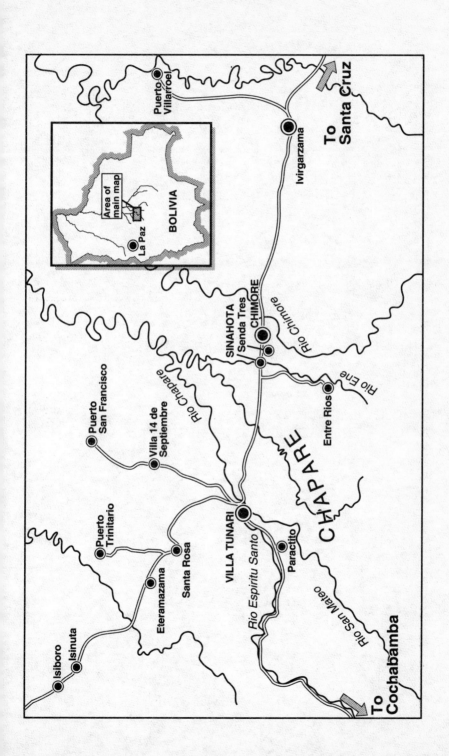

Introduction

ONE chill day in July 1991, Pablo Escobar, the godfather of Colombia's notorious Medellín cocaine cartel, quietly surrendered to the authorities. He handed his pistol to officials on the outskirts of Medellín and was whisked by helicopter to a special prison in the Andean foothills overlooking his boyhood town of Envigado. After nearly a year on the run, the world's Number One cocaine boss had chosen the day and the conditions of his surrender and imprisonment. Some thought the ranch-style prison camp was more like a five-star hotel: spread over ten acres, it had its own soccer field, a king-size bed and furnishings handpicked by the chubby-faced multi-billionaire himself. A 5000-volt electric fence reinforced with barbed wire circled the camp, but it was not so much to keep the druglord in as to keep his enemies out. None the less officials hailed the imprisonment of the world's most wanted man as a turning point in the world-wide war against cocaine.

In fact, Escobar's incarceration was not quite the victory it seemed. From 1989 when the Colombian government declared all-out war on the drug cartels and US President Bush put the fight against cocaine top of his agenda, the rival Cali cartel had been quietly taking the upper hand. Medellín cartel members had spread their smuggling and cocaine processing operations to nearly a dozen other Latin American nations. They joined cocaine barons in those countries who were silently building up their empires while international attention focused on Colombia.

One of the cocaine trade's most important new centres is Bolivia, a landlocked country of gaunt snow-capped Andean mountains and semi-tropical jungle lowlands. The poorest nation in South America, it is also the most cocaine-addicted. Cocaine exports outstrip legal exports, around one in five Bolivians work in cocaine-related jobs and without cocaine the country's economy would collapse. In 1980 drug traffickers managed to install their own government in a military takeover which became known as the 'cocaine coup'. In 1984, the country's Number One drug boss, Roberto Suárez, was so powerful he offered to pay off the foreign debt.

Bolivian Indians have cultivated the coca leaf, the raw material for cocaine, on the steamy eastern slopes of the Andes for thousands of years. It is chewed by inhabitants of the highlands to make life a little more tolerable and is used too as a medicine. Today Bolivia is the second largest producer of coca leaf after Peru and produces roughly a third of the world supply.

Whereas in the past Bolivia confined itself to growing leaves, it has now also become one of the world's largest manufacturers of finished cocaine. The process began in the early 1980s but was speeded up by the Colombian clamp-down in 1989. Bolivian traffickers, who previously sold their partly manufactured cocaine to Colombians to process further, had no-one to sell to and were forced to do it themselves. From 1989 to 1991 production of finished cocaine in Bolivia tripled. In 1990 Bolivia made at least 200 tonnes of the stuff, making it the second largest producer in the world after Colombia. Soon, drug experts believe, it could become the largest.

The Colombian crack-down had another disturbing effect. Export routes to the United States via Colombia were disrupted, so South American countries like Bolivia began to export to Europe. In any case, the US market was nearing saturation. Europe, including Britain, was targeted as the growth market of the future. As one Interpol agent who is studying the expansion of cocaine into Europe remarked in the middle of the 1991 recession, 'We must be among the few people who are at absolutely no risk of being made unemployed.'

This book looks at Bolivia. Unlike previous books on the cocaine trade which tend to look at the problem through Western eyes, this one looks at the drugs business through the eyes of the main players in the country where the white powder is made: from coca farmers, to drug barons, to the military, to politicians. Each shows how the profits to be made from cocaine are as addictive as the drug itself and how, without a drastic drop in demand from the West, the prospects of weaning Bolivia off cocaine are minimal. The book also looks at Western anti-drug policies. It asks whether they are effective or whether, in some cases, they are actually counter productive.

Finally, some words of caution. Because the cocaine industry is illegal, manufacturers do not produce balance sheets or end of year results. Officials may guess how much cocaine is made, but nobody knows the real amount. Estimates of production of finished cocaine, for example, are based on satellite pictures of coca fields or on seizures (Customs in Britain, for example, estimate they seize around 10 per cent of the amount actually in circulation). But the resulting figures rarely tally and can vary wildly. Estimates of how much coca is grown in Bolivia, for example, range from 50,000 hectares to double that amount. All estimates quoted in this book must therefore be treated as 'guesstimates'. Another problem is that governments manipulate the figures to suit their political needs. Andean governments, for instance, tend to err on the generous side when estimating coca production in order to gain more aid. The United States, on the other hand, tends to play it down so as to show it is winning its 'war on drugs.'

Similar caution should be applied to much of the information in this book. In a country as hooked on cocaine as Bolivia, it is often difficult to know the real interests of interviewees, however sincere they may appear. Little, in the underworld of drugs, is what it seems. Almost all the information in this book is based on my own interviews and wherever possible is corroborated by other sources. I have identified sources as fully as possible and tried to avoid use of unnamed ones. Many Bolivian officials have provided information at considerable risk to their lives and careers. When, however, for security reasons, they have requested anonymity, I have respected their wishes.

The cocaine business, and efforts to thwart it, are also changing all the time. The price of the coca leaf fluctuates daily. Druglords get arrested or give themselves up while new ones fill their shoes. Manufacturing methods and export routes change as the result of law enforcement efforts. The information in this book is up to date at the time of completion (September 1991), but it is inevitable that some details and names will have changed by the time it is published.

Some readers may be surprised that this book does not offer solutions. Numerous other books and articles have attempted to do that. The aim of this book is to show what is, rather than what might be. It is about the realities of the everyday lives of the people involved in the drugs trade, whether participating in it or fighting it, and the dilemmas they face. Hopefully the reader will draw her or his own conclusions.

1

The Ultimate High:
The Consumers

My name is Rob. I was 11 when I first started drugs. We lived in a block of flats called Potomac Gardens on I Street in southeast Washington DC. My dad was using drugs and abused me and my mother regularly. He beat me with an old slipper when he was angry. I also had an infection in my left ear. It oozed this horrible yellow liquid. It smelt real bad. People used to talk about me at school and make fun of me. I wanted to block it out, get away from the pain, so I used drugs. It was marijuana then. I stole it from the stash at home.

As I started to use drugs, I got addicted. At first it was escaping reality, it was a fun and pleasure thing. Then it wasn't fun any more. I started looking for new drugs, anything that would change my mood.

I remember the first time I snorted cocaine. I was 14. I felt light headed, rejuvenated, as if I'd got a full tank of gas. I could smell everything, the flowers, the trees. The high lasted about two hours. At that time I didn't have to buy the cocaine. Friends just gave it to me. 'Go on, try it,' they said. I wanted to be part of the crowd, I wanted them to look up to me and say 'Hey, he's used cocaine'. So I did it. We used it together in a house, a car, outside, anywhere.

Cocaine was a drug that people liked to have fun with. People were impressed, they thought it was flashy. Girls clung to me. It was like another asset, like a fast car. Even when I said 'No' people still gave me dope. I was soon addicted but I didn't realise it. I was enjoying myself. Sometimes it was rough, but when I was high, nothing mattered. I had no feeling whether I was sad or happy. I didn't care. Everyone was doing drugs.

1

Sometimes I liked speedballing, mixing cocaine with heroin. Cocaine made me speed, heroin made me nod. It gave me a nice level high.

By now I was hitting regular. Every morning when I woke up, before thinking about eating, even going to the bathroom, I had to get it in me, just to feel natural. Otherwise I'd feel physically sick. I stopped eating. My weight dropped to 136 pounds from my normal 206. I looked terrible. At night I couldn't sleep. When I stopped bingeing, I got depressed and irritable so had to use more.

Other parts of my life began to get out of hand. I worked as a clerk typist at Federal Communications but I lost my job. I was also studying at University of DC for a degree in Computer Systems but soon that went down the tube too. I began to turn up three days a week, then two days. Then just weekends, then no days at all. The drugs stopped me seeing that my life was screwed up. All I could see was that I needed cocaine.

I was spending between $100 and $160 a week on drugs. I was using so heavy I couldn't pay for my classes no more or rather, I could have, but my addiction wouldn't let me. The fees were $500 a semester and I could have afforded it. But instead I wanted $90 Nike shoes, $50 shirts — and dope.

I would do anything to get the money to satisfy my craving. Sometimes I sold dope to get money. I sold heroin, coke, PCP, crack, anything, in houses, on the streets. I even sold to children. They were 16, 17, sometimes 11, elementary school kids. But I didn't care. All I cared about was getting the finances I needed. Some people I knew got so desperate they'd even sell their kids for an ounce of coke.

Other times I ran out of money I just went stealing from people's houses. I liked getting in, roaming around, doing what I had to do. Then I'd sell the stuff easy. Sometimes I sold it to the dope man himself. Others guys stole from their friends, from their parents. The girls just sold their bodies.

With girls I was just fulfilling my needs. I was seeking love and attention that I hadn't had as a child. I had to have at least three girls a day. If they were nice girls from nice families I didn't get high with them. I missed so much in terms of living. When you are on drugs you can't love anybody. I was just falling, doing devilish things. Drugs take the reality out of your life. In real life a person has to be responsible for their actions and has to do things as an adult. Drugs take that away from you, they have you living a false life. All you can see is the people that's out there on the street corners in their sweatshirts, their gold chains, their BMWs. I couldn't see it was all a web of illusion.

CALL it snow, white lady, Charlie, toot, happy dust, flake, nose candy, C, blow, or simply coke. Whatever name you give it, cocaine has become America's favourite drug. Since the early 1980s it has swept the country like a white blizzard, leaving a trail of shattered lives, 'crack babies' and street-gang violence. Once considered the 'champagne' of drugs, consumed by the glittering Hollywood jet set, cocaine, in its smokeable form of crack, now provides an illusion of comfort to the drop-outs and unemployed of America's impoverished inner cities. 'We are facing an epidemic that is out of control,' warned Senator Joseph Biden, chairman of a US senate committee on drugs, in 1990. 'Unless we take decisive action to fight the crisis, our streets and schools will never be safe, and a large part of this generation of Americans will be lost.'[1]

He was not exaggerating. Americans consume more cocaine than any other industrialised country. Over 22 million say they have tried the harmless-looking white powder and between two and three million are addicted to it. In 1989, around 2,500 Americans who 'just said Yes' died of cocaine-related causes. In 1990, one in five people arrested for any crime were found to be hooked on cocaine or crack. Americans spend a staggering $110,000 million a year on drugs ($28,000 million on cocaine), more than double the profits of all the Fortune 500 companies put together and the equivalent of America's entire gross agricultural income. Drug use is costing over $100,000 million in lost productivity and drug-related accidents.

Today cocaine, in the form of crack, is associated with the poverty and violence of America's 'underclass'. But it was not always so. When it first became fashionable in the early 1980s it was the sinful secret of Hollywood film stars and Wall Street whizz kids who snorted it from coffee tables through crisp rolled-up $100 notes. Seen as a symbol of wealth and status, coke became the drug of choice for millions of conventional and upwardly mobile wealthy Americans, from lawyers to businessmen to government bureaucrats and politicians. It made them talkative and gave them the illusion of being able to cope in stressful environments. Since cocaine, at over $100 a gramme, was the vice of the respectable rich, the police rarely interfered.

The view that coke was glamorous, harmless and socially acceptable was typified in a now famous, or infamous, article in *Time* magazine in July 1981. 'A snort in each nostril and you're up and away for 30 minutes or so,' the article said. 'Alert, witty and with it. No hangover. No physical addiction. No lung cancer.... Instead, drive, sparkle, energy.' It quoted Robert Sabbag, the author of a 1976 study of cocaine called *Snowblind*, who said that 'Cocaine, like motorcycles, machine guns and White House politics is, among many things, a virility substitute. Its mere possession imparts status: cocaine equals money, and money equals power.'[2]

Time quoted cooks at a restaurant near Boston, who celebrated the last day of their work week as Coke Day, sniffing the white powder from their first order to their last, joined by dishwashers and waiters who popped by for an occasional hit. Another group of young professionals in Pasadena, California, celebrated TGIW (Thank God It's Wednesday) by gathering at the home of a local car dealer for a coke session at cocktail time.

Coke had a place in business too. Maids who worked at condominiums in Aspen, Colorado, found little piles of cocaine left as tips on the table when they went to clean. The town was known as Toot City because it had so much cocaine. Others used the drug as a barter item, exchanging grammes or 'quarters' for dental treatment, accountancy fees or a discount on a new car. In Madison Avenue, New York, ad men offered clients coke instead of martinis. Said one advertising executive: 'Spill out a couple of grammes of that white stuff on the table and everyone knows where you're coming from.'

The magazine gave graphic descriptions of 'head shops', like Lady Snow's in Hollywood, which sold coke paraphernalia. There were gleaming jade cutting stones, gold razor blades to chop coke crystals and tiny brown bottles for sniffing. One Iranian had paid $28,000 for an antique gold Tiffany snuff bottle capable of holding two grammes of cocaine. There were silver sniffing-spoons which users could flaunt on chains around their necks.

Then suddenly in the mid-1980s the price of cocaine began to plummet. The South American countries that grew the coca leaf (the raw material for cocaine) and processed it into cocaine had woken up to the huge demand from the north and were now flooding the US market. Between 1982 and 1988 the wholesale price of cocaine fell from around $60,000 to about $25,000 a kilo. Cocaine became so cheap that ordinary Americans could now share what had previously been an exotic indulgence of the affluent.

The biggest revolution was the appearance of crack. Unlike cocaine powder, which was snorted or sniffed, crack was smoked, or 'free based'. Since smoking was the most direct route to the brain, it hit the nervous system like a jackhammer, inducing instant euphoria. Crack's greatest significance was that it was priced within reach of the very young and the poor. A vial of crack could be bought on the streets for $5 to $10, little more than the cost of a cinema ticket.

The other secret of crack's success was that anybody could make it. All you need is a kitchen. And the recipe is as easy as any out of *Good House-keeping*: 'Take two ounces of cocaine hydrochloride [cocaine powder]. Mix with two ounces of comeback [a chemical adulterant] and one ounce of bicarbonate of soda. Add water and slowly bring to the boil. Allow to cool into a solid mass then "crack" into rock-like segments. Smoke. Intense rush should follow instantly. Serves 2,000.'

The raisin-sized off-white chunks, known as 'rocks', which look like soap shavings or teeth, are sold on the streets in packets or vials, or sometimes in three-inch sticks with ridges, referred to as 'french fries' or 'teeth'. Crack, which gets its name from the sound it makes when smoked, is inhaled through homemade 'pipes', or through cigarettes.

Cocaine (in the form of crack) did best where Americans did worst. Whereas cocaine had been the 'champagne drug', crack was the 'losers' drug'. Underclass Americans turned to crack as an escape from sterile poverty, child abuse or marital problems. Dealers, mostly impoverished Dominican and Jamaican immigrants, cashed in, setting up open air 'crack markets' in dreary inner city estates. They set up outlets outside schools, enticing teenagers with free samples, or waited outside welfare offices for single mothers who had just collected their fortnightly payments. Gangs (or 'crews') in expensive Nike shoes and gold chains patrolled their turfs with M-16s and jackknives, fighting 'crack wars' among themselves when supplies outstripped clients. As cocaine-related crime spiralled, Washington DC won the dubious reputation as murder capital of the US.

Crack's effect on the US has been catastrophic. Babies born to crack-addicted mothers (300,000 of them in 1990) suffer from birth defects like malformed kidneys and genitals. In 1988 the *Washington Post* reported that one in five women giving birth at Washington General Hospital was using drugs. Crack is bankrupting families, shattering marriages and destroying the social fabric of inner city neighbourhoods all over the US. Worst of all, crackheads will do anything to keep their habit going. Having depleted their bank accounts, they rob their families, sell their cars, businesses and even their children. Some spend as much as $1,000 a week. When the money runs out, many turn to crime. 'We have never dealt with a drug that has caused people to resort to violence the way that crack does,' says John Wilder, former head of the Washington division of the US Drug Enforcement Administration. 'With other drugs we knew what to expect when we went to the door. Today it's different. It's not one gun, or a common six-shooter gun, it's normally a street sweeper, like an old tommy gun with shotgun shells. Its only purpose is to kill a lot of people. Crack is such a devastating drug that people don't have any second thoughts about killing, simply because of what it does to the mind and the body.' Now, says Wilder, DEA and FBI agents carry semi-automatic hand-guns and wear bullet-proof vests when they raid 'crackhouses'.[3]

With the rise of crack, many middle-class Americans began to turn against drugs, adhering to the philosophy of 'zero tolerance' fostered by the Reagan administration. In reality, though, the image of crack as an 'underclass' inner-city drug is only partially true. Although their resources make it easier to keep their habit secret, significant numbers of white, affluent and middle-income Americans are addicted. Dr Arnold Washton, the director of a New York treatment centre, says around 70 per cent of the addicts he treats are middle-class people with good jobs. 'These new addicts are business executives and... doctors and receptionists. And if you met them on the street or at the Little League game, you wouldn't have a clue they're smoking their brains out on crack back home in the basement.... Crack is definitely an equal opportunity drug.' Dr Rosescan, who heads the cocaine

abuse centre at New York's Columbia-Presbyterian Medical Centre, says '[Crack] is proving to be just as addictive among the middle class. Only it's more behind closed doors in nice homes.'[4]

In 1990, the *New York Times*[5] told the story of 37-year-old Mary G, who realised what had happened to her life during a row with her husband. He was complaining about the messy apartment and lack of dinner again when their four-year-old daughter rose to her mother's defence. 'Daddy, Daddy, Mommy's OK as long as she has her pipe.'

Mary had first started smoking marijuana when she was 12 and later moved on to cocaine. She gave up everything when the child was born. But as soon as she was weaned, Mary returned to crack. 'I said, "Hey, I can handle this."' But once a week became twice a week and then three and four times. Mary would drop her daughter off at nursery school, go to a friend's apartment, smoke crack all day and pick her daughter up at 5.30. 'I told myself it was OK as long as I didn't take crack home,' Mary said. 'I'd make dinner, give my daughter a bath, read her stories and put her to bed. Then when my husband fell asleep, I'd go to a cash machine, get some money and find a street dealer so I could smoke it in the bathroom.'

Mary became so eager to reach her friend's apartment and begin smoking crack that she would not bother to stop and leave her daughter at the school but would take her along too. 'She saw me crawling around on that floor looking for little pieces of crack, as if it was gold. I could have given up my husband, my daughter, my whole life and crawled into that pipe. I was so disgusting. We in the middle class can get away with so much more. We're not robbing stores. We just steal from ourselves and our families.'

Between 1984 and 1989 use of cocaine and crack soared. The number of Americans admitted to hospital emergency rooms as a result of using cocaine increased more than five times. Deaths from cocaine-related causes more than doubled (although illegal drugs still cannot compete as killers with their legal equivalents, tobacco and alcohol). In 1989 alone, nearly 2,500 Americans died as a result of cocaine abuse.[6]

Cocaine is one of the most powerful stimulants known to humankind. Unlike heroin, which is a depressant, cocaine stimulates the body's natural response to pleasure, creating a feeling of euphoria and power. A Manhattan ballerina who used cocaine described her experience: 'It makes you shiver in tune with the raw, volcanic energy of New York. It bleeds your senses till you see the city as an epileptic rainbow, trembling at the speed of light.'

In contrast with cocaine, which takes up to five minutes to have an effect, crack acts on the brain almost immediately, producing an instant intense 'rush' ten times stronger than the effect of cocaine. The rush is also briefer. The high from cocaine may last 15 to 30 minutes. With crack it rarely lasts ten, and is followed by an intense low which leaves the user craving more. 'Cocaine is like sitting down and feeling you're going 500 miles an hour,' says Eric, a former addict. 'Crack is completely different, it's like an astronaut floating in space.' Dr Frank Gawin, a leading US expert, calls crack 'the most intense euphoria we know about'.

The after-effects of cocaine and crack are less euphoric. High doses can damage the brain, causing violent, erratic or paranoid behaviour, and over-strain the heart, leading to cardiac arrest. Some users develop psychoses, hearing or seeing things that do not exist, or experiencing 'coke bugs' — feeling that hundreds of insects are crawling out of their skin. In the long term, users may develop heart problems and digestive disorders and become impotent.

None the less, many of those who used cocaine in the 1970s did so in the belief that it was 'safe' and non-addictive. Such beliefs collapsed when prominent US figures like the actor John Belushi and the basketball star Len Bias died of overdoses. Some US experts claim cocaine (and particularly crack) is one of the world's most addictive drugs. They estimate that around one in ten people who start using cocaine 'recreationally' will go on to serious, heavy use, and say it is impossible for users to predict or control the extent to which they use the drug. Other experts disagree, pointing out that many users take cocaine for years and never become addicted. They say cocaine is far less physically addictive than heroin, although they admit that the psychological craving for the good feelings experienced on a high may have the same effect of dependence. Ironically, in 1975 a US Domestic Council Drug Abuse Task Force chaired by Vice-President Nelson Rockefeller produced a white paper which stated that 'cocaine is not physically addictive'.

The debate is even more intense over the addictiveness of crack. Many experts claim it is instantly addictive, making occasional use impossible. This is disputed by studies like a 1988 survey of 308 adolescent drug users in Miami, which showed that although over 90 per cent had tried crack, only 29 per cent used it daily and then only one or two hits at a time.[7] Another US survey of drug dependent teenagers showed that heavy crack users took three months to begin using it even on a weekly basis.[8] Addiction to cocaine, it estimated, would take longer, probably several months.

As cocaine swept the US, social scientists tried to explain why the US is so far ahead of other industrial countries in terms of drug use. 'This is a country where crimes that produce income are unusually rewarding,' says Mark Kleiman, a lecturer in public policy at Harvard University's John F. Kennedy School of Government and formerly a senior Justice Department official responsible for drug policy.[9] 'The class system here is less confining than in Europe and there's enough geographic and social mobility that a person who makes big money from crime can really move up the scale.' Others attribute the epidemic to social problems and a breakdown in law enforcement in inner cities. For those whose lives are empty, crack and cocaine provide temporary highs. 'What is new' says Stanton Peele, a psychologist with Mathematica Policy Research Inc., 'is [the] large numbers of inner city people, blacks and Hispanics, [with] a real level of hopelessness. Most northern European countries have nothing remotely comparable.'[10]

THEY MAY have nothing comparable, but Europe is not immune to the deadly white wave sweeping America. Both availability and use of cocaine are rising fast and, according to some intelligence experts, could soon reach US levels. Between 1989 and 1990 the amount of cocaine confiscated in Europe more than doubled, from 6 to 14 tonnes. Given that police estimate they seize a maximum of 10 per cent of the total, that means that in 1990 Europe was awash with at least 140 tonnes of snow.

Drug enforcement officials think they know why: South American drug barons have seen their outlets to North America squeezed by law enforcement and oversupply, and are looking for new markets. While Colombian police have targeted the Medellín cartel, for example, the rival Cali cartel has been quietly intensifying its efforts to make Europe the growth market of the 1990s. Cali now reportedly supplies around 90 per cent of Europe's coke. Bolivian and Peruvian traffickers are also exporting directly to Europe. 'We are no longer seeing as much of the north-south movement,' says Raymond Kendall, Interpol's executive director. 'Traffickers are switching from Caribbean routes to new ones through Brazil's Amazon waterways and Argentina through Africa and Europe's major ports.' One US drug enforcement official calculates that as much as 40 per cent of world cocaine supply goes to Europe, compared to 60 per cent to the US. By 2000, he guesses, the percentages will be the other way round. 'The next ten years are going to be exciting in Europe,' says Joe Toft, a Drug Enforcement Administration official in Bogotá. 'But they are also going to be tough. This decade could be more like a nightmare than a dream.' Robert Bonner, the Administration's head, is even more forceful. 'It may take two or three years before you see the full, devastating effects cocaine causes,' he warned UK officials in December 1991. 'But it is almost as certain as night follows day that it will happen unless effective measures are taken.'

Although the risks and costs of getting cocaine to Europe are greater, the prices make it worthwhile. A kilo, which fetches a mere $12,000 to $15,000 in Miami, can fetch three to four times that in Europe. South American drug barons now have networks in virtually every European country and are joining forces with home-grown mafia like the Italian Mafia. According to Italian intelligence reports, the Mafia has forced the Colombians into a 'business relationship' by threatening to eliminate any cocaine couriers who operate without their blessing.

The druglords are also making tentative inroads into Japan, where the going wholesale price is as high as $65,000 a kilo. In 1990 an estimated 69 kilos entered Japan, five times more than the year before, and there are growing signs that *yakuza* gangsters are liaising with South American drug barons to expand imports dramatically over the next few years. A report by members of the European Parliament in 1991 voiced fears that Japanese businesses moving into Europe will bring the *yakuza*, known to be well connected with top Japanese companies, with them. A white paper by Japan's National Police Agency warned that if nothing were done quickly to stop the trend, Japan's drug problem would soon match that of the US. 'With little awareness over cocaine and the fact that gangsters are expanding their drug business with South American traffickers, there is a real danger that cocaine and other drug usage will spread throughout Japan.'

In Europe, Latin druglords are preparing to exploit the dismantling of internal frontier controls after 1992 following the formation of a single European Market. The removal of barriers is worrying customs officials, particularly in Britain. They hope to compensate by increasing intelligence gathering, improving cooperation between police in member states and tightening land, air and sea controls on the EC's external borders. A European Drugs Intelligence Unit was due to be set up in 1992, staffed by police and customs officials from member states and drug liaison officers from key non-member states, to enable national agencies to pool information and coordinate their efforts for the first time. British customs officials say they will maintain checks on vehicles, aircraft and ships which other European countries will do away with.

Spain, with its historical and linguistic ties with South America, is the main entry point into Europe. In 1991 Spanish police fished more than 1,300 kilos out of the Atlantic. Smugglers had hidden it on the craggy Galician coast to collect later but a storm set dozens of 30-kilo packages adrift. In another incident, police seized a boat loaded with one tonne of Colombian cocaine. Still more worrying, they later discovered that cocaine worth nearly $300 million had been smuggled into Spain by Pablo Escobar's Medellín cartel despite the fact that the drug boss was in gaol.

Another target is The Netherlands where container ships carrying drugs have a good chance of passing unnoticed among the 7,000 that enter Rotterdam every day. Cocaine smugglers also like The Netherlands because they believe they will be treated leniently if caught. In 1990 Dutch officials seized a load of nearly three tons of Cali coke hidden in drums of passionfruit juice on a Swiss-flag freighter. 'It was the biggest confiscation of drugs in Europe and an indication that the days of the occasional kilo are over. Now we are in the age of the occasional ton of cocaine,' says an agent. The Netherlands is also used as a storage depot from where cocaine is shipped to other destinations, including Britain.

Increasing amounts of cocaine are passing through former Eastern bloc countries which lack sophisticated customs networks. 'This is a weak point for anti-drugs arrangements,' says a customs official. 'You have a reasonable chance of not being caught.' Police forces there are demoralised by political upheaval, borders have been pulled open, and criminal groups are already in place. Laundering of profits from drug smuggling is also likely to become an increasing problem as previously inconvertible currencies harden and become attractive to traffickers. 'Since the revolutions in Central and Eastern Europe,' said Britain's Home Office Minister John Patten, 'there has been a massive increase in the flow of goods and people across borders. This freedom of movement, while very welcome in itself, has provided greater opportunities for drug traffickers.' As yet, there is no domestic market in former Eastern bloc countries, as people are still too poor to afford drugs.

In Britain, cocaine has already caught up with the country's traditional problem drug, heroin. In 1990, 605 kilos were seized, 32 per cent more than in 1989. By the end of the first half of 1991, 625 kilos had already been seized, boosted by a record haul of half a ton from a freighter in Ullapool, northwest Scotland. Some customs officers believed the size of the shipment showed that South American traffickers, under increasing pressure in the US and in Colombia, were dumping their produce on Britain.

Only a small percentage reaches Britain direct. South American traffickers do not have the family or criminal links they have with countries like Spain, and many do not speak English. 'South Americans tend to steer clear of Britain. They feel uncomfortable,' says a customs officer. 'They are afraid of the British police and the penalties are severe.'

Most cocaine reaches Britain via third countries, mostly in Europe, but also in Africa, like Nigeria. In Spain and The Netherlands distribution is carried out by gangs of expatriate Britons who have years of experience dealing in marijuana. Some cocaine is sent from Jamaica or the US by sophisticated 'yardie' gangs or 'posses' who link up with similar gangs in Britain. It is carried kilo by kilo by couriers, usually young West Indian single mothers, who strap it to their bodies and run the customs gauntlet at Heathrow.

Britain's cocaine market is still centred predominantly around London and the southeast, although experts believe there is also a developing market in the northwest, in areas like Merseyside and Manchester, and in Birmingham. It sells at between £40 and £60 a gramme, depending on whether the buyer is 'connected', but purity varies widely, diminishing as it moves away from London. Because public attention has until now focused almost exclusively on heroin, no-one really knows the extent of the coke problem. Police and social workers say users straddle class boundaries, and range from high-achieving City businessmen and media stars to inhabitants of deprived inner city areas like Brixton, south London, and Harlesden in northwest London. In east London, many are white working-class Thatcherites who worked their way up from barrow boys to dealers in the City. 'They are part of the yuppie culture,' says Viv Reid, director of the Newham Drugs Advice Centre, which specialises in treating and helping cocaine users.

In contrast to heroin, which is a 'getting away from it all' drug, cocaine is seen as a 'being-on-top' drug, Reid says. 'You take cocaine because you want to be a player, to be the best, to be confident.' One of Reid's typical clients is a stockbroker who earns £50,000 basic salary, plus £80,000 in commissions.

> He has cocaine delivered to his office by courtesy services who enclose it with sandwiches or coke. He can't relax at the end of the day, so he snorts some coke and stays in a hotel with a prostitute. He never sees his wife and family. If his suit is dirty next morning, he buys a new one. If you have the money, cocaine is seen as socially acceptable. You are unlikely to have any problems at first and if you have money you can get help from a private clinic. The problems start when you run out of money and you stop dealing. You get stressed out and paranoid. People come to us when they're desperate and down to the last of four houses.

Given the US experience, in the late 1980s many experts predicted that cocaine use in Britain would explode into a crack epidemic. In 1989 a US Drug Enforcement Administration agent called Robert Stutman gave his 'personal guarantee' that within two years Britain would have a crack problem almost as serious as that of the US. Douglas Hurd, then Home Secretary, was so concerned that he called a special meeting of the Pompidou Group of European ministers at which he compared crack to a medieval plague menacing Europe. Douglas Hogg, then minister of state at the Home Office, made a tour of Washington DC's grimy crack-ridden streets to see the problem for himself. A police crack unit was set up, and customs and police established a joint crack task-force to tackle courier traffic across the Atlantic.

In fact, the explosion did not happen, at least not when predicted. In 1990 the police seized less than one kilo of crack in the whole of Britain, virtually all of it in London, though it must be said that was over three times the amount seized the previous year. Some believed there was no reason why Britain should follow the US path. Crack had been sold in The Netherlands since 1973, for example, but had never caught on. Britain also has a better intelligence network than the US, and totally different social and economic conditions. Also, since the Kray brothers were put behind bars in 1969, police claim that Britain no longer has the organised criminal gangs to distribute crack. Distributors work as individuals who give one another a hand when they have to supply a big order. It is safer that way. 'They are not an organisation with a hierarchy,' says Detective Chief Superintendent Derek Todd, chief of Scotland Yard's drugs squad. 'A guy may be top one day, but when he goes to gaol he's nothing.'

None the less, there are definite signs that crack, or rock as it is known on the street, is on the increase and could soon become an epidemic. When crack first arrived in about 1988 police raids uncovered between 20 and 30 rocks. Now they find between 100 and 200. In May 1991 police made their biggest ever haul when they seized around a kilo of crack, worth more than £500,000, in northwest London, more than the previous year's total seizures.

Although most of those arrested for crack abuse are black, treatment centres say users are divided more or less equally between blacks and whites. Most graduate to rock from cocaine. Reid says that 'wash rock' (so called because it has been 'washed' or processed) is often preferred because it is seen as 'cleaner', 'better for you'. Although the cheapest way to obtain rock is to make it oneself, many users are unwilling to go through the bother of 'washing up' and prefer to 'eat' (smoke), he says. First-time users are offered free samples by dealers eager to win new customers. After that rocks can cost anything from £5 to £100, depending on their size. Average users spend around £500 a week, but some blow as much as £2,000. Like cocaine, crack gives them a sense of power, of being on top. Women use rock to help them perform sexually; like Paula, who buys ten rocks a day and has a man for each.

Many dealers start selling in order to pay for their user habit. After a while some become so paranoid they do business alone on the phone at home and sleep with a shotgun. Like their US counterparts, British dealers never keep drugs on them or in their homes, storing them instead in stashes on areas of waste ground or in 'safe houses'. Police say dealers are predominantly blacks and 'yardies', although people in crack-user communities claim this is misleading and that, like users, dealers are divided more or less equally between blacks and whites. They say police focus on blacks because blacks are less professional and more ostentatious with their wealth and therefore more visible.

In east London and Essex, distribution is run by white criminal families who have controlled the streets for generations and already deal in speed, acid and heroin. They have the distribution networks, and the links with the police who are often from the same families and drink in the same pubs. They sell to intermediaries, black or white, who distribute to their various communities. Because of their experience, the white East End dealers know how to avoid the eye of the police: they rarely do business on the street, preferring to use networks of friends and family; they shun shootouts which only draw attention; and they front their wealth by buying small businesses. 'The first thing a white dealer does when he starts up is fork out two or three hundred quid to buy a scanner to monitor the police,' says Reid.

Black dealers, by contrast, don't bother, says Reid. They like to spend their money and deal openly on the streets. New to the business, they are still seduced by the image of gun-toting *Miami Vice* style cowboys who know no fear. 'They want women, fast cars, expensive clothes,' says Reid.

They may carry £50,000-worth of assets on themselves, like gold chains and rings and designer clothes. The white dealers wear Italian sports clothes which you don't know are expensive unless you look at the label, but the blacks wear clothes that are blatantly designer made. In an area like Notting Hill, you can see lines of Mercedes parked on the roadsides. I even know one 13-year-old who bought himself a £30,000 Merc. Black dealers also attract police attention by their use of

Mafia-style shootouts. Whites prefer to remove someone quietly, make him 'disappear'.

Crack-linked violence may be increasing. In May 1991 a police officer was seriously wounded after being shot at with a .32 Colt automatic. Police say more and more dealers appear to be using weapons to fight for territory and a corner in a highly lucrative and increasingly competitive business. Getting hold of guns, which double up as status symbols, is easy. 'You just pass the word that you want a gun, and someone will get one for you,' says Reid. 'One man I knew had 20 brand new hand-guns with ammunition that he was trying to sell.'

The crack epidemic may simply be reaching Britain a little later than expected. 'The crack boom didn't happen when it was predicted. But the signs are that it's happening now,' says Detective Chief Superintendent Roger Stoodley, who carried out an inquiry into organised crime in 1991. 'The baby needs time to grow,' says Reid. 'But in some areas, like parts of south and west London, the epidemic is already here.'

If that is true, Britain is not ready. Having focused for years on treating heroin junkies, drug treatment agencies do not have facilities to cope with cocaine and crack addicts, whose needs and outlook are completely different. The biggest problem is getting users to seek treatment in the first place. Whereas heroin addicts may seek help after weeks, it can take years for a rock addict to go to a centre. 'They have to be at the end of their tether before they admit they have a problem,' says Reid. When they arrive at a centre, they can be difficult customers. 'These are strong people, they like taking the piss. They can leave workers at the centres feeling deskilled.' They also refuse to associate with heroin junkies, whom they see as anti-social, smelly, and AIDS-ridden. And cocaine addiction is even more difficult to treat. Heroin addicts have been weaned off their addiction with a methadone substitute but no substitute has yet been found for cocaine.

AT 9.00 p.m. eastern time on 5 September 1989, a grim-faced President Bush appeared on US television to make his first prime time address to the nation. The speech was to deal with a subject that ranked top in the collective mind of the US public — drugs — and he was to outline a brand new strategy on how to fight them. His publicity agents were determined to make it a theatrical occasion. Administration officials had been grooming the media for weeks, whetting their appetites with advance morsels. Bush had practised the speech, which had been rewritten several times, for an hour in the morning and 45 minutes in the afternoon with his campaign news media adviser.

Bush's words, when he spoke, were those of a man ready for battle. 'Drugs are sapping our strength as a nation', he declared. 'There is no match for a united America, a determined America, an angry America. Our outrage against drugs unites us, brings us together behind this one plan of action, an assault on every front.' In the course of his speech the US president used the word 'fight' 11 times, 'war' and 'threat' each four times, 'battle' and 'victory' twice.

In the sixth paragraph, Bush kept up the theatrical mood by holding up a small plastic bag as gingerly as if it were a urine specimen. 'This is crack cocaine,' he said earnestly, 'seized a few days ago by Drug Enforcement Administration agents in Lafayette Park just across the street from the White House. It's as innocent looking as candy, but it's turning our cities into battle zones and is murdering our children. But let there be no mistake. This stuff is poison.' What he did not let on was the considerable lengths to which the Drug Enforcement Agency (DEA) had had to go to get hold of the stage prop. Bush's speech writers had had to get the police to stage a 'buy' specially to make the point about how the terrible sea of drugs was lapping at the sacred shores of the White House. They had had to stage it because the park, heavily patrolled by Secret Service and police, happened to be one of the few cocaine-free spots in Washington. In fact the sale had been notoriously tricky to arrange because the dealer in question had never heard of the White House, did not know how to find it on the map and was baffled why anyone would want to make such complicated plans just to buy a few rocks of low-grade crack.

When faced with a particularly intractable problem or flagging popular support, US presidents have a favourite solution: declare war. For Carter it was the oil crisis; for Reagan the Red Menace; for Bush it is drugs and, most recently, Saddam Hussein. The US, it seems, does not feel happy unless it has a war of some kind to fight. War gives it a sense of moral purpose, of strength on the world stage. When 1989 opinion polls showed that the US public viewed drugs as the most dangerous problem confronting the country, politicians realised they had to look as if they were doing something, and doing it tough, if they wanted to stick around.

Wars, however, need enemies. And enemies, almost by definition, need to live outside the country. Like the Red Menace, the White Menace is likened to a plague threatening innocent Americans. Unless they fight back, more and more will be smitten, like catching measles or the flu. Others compare the drugs menace to a military invasion. As congressman Stephen Solarz put it: 'If intercontinental ballistic missiles were being fired on US cities from Peru and Bolivia, surely our government would have devised a plan to knock out the enemy. Why then should we treat the threat posed by the international cartels so lightly?'[11]

Such images portray the South American countries that produce cocaine (Peru, Colombia and Bolivia) as the root of the problem. Although Bush has claimed publicly that US demand is as much to blame as South American supply, US policies are still driven by the belief that it is the aggressive invasion of the US by cheap Andean coke that has driven so many young

Americans to become addicted, not their own shortcomings. As *Newsweek* put it in 1988: 'America's cocaine problem... has been caused by the Colombian cartels and their US-based accomplices.... America has no choice: it must begin to fight back.'[12] Congressmen in particular have used inflated rhetoric to rail against the 'external' threat. Even though privately some have reservations about the morality and practicality of a strategy that targets producer rather than consumer countries, in public they are vociferous in blaming Andean nations, correctly viewing this as an easy way to make political capital without having to produce immediate results at home. Furthermore, by blaming the South Americans for the drug problem, the social, political and environmental costs of controlling it are borne by them, rather than by North Americans. Policies that would be unacceptable at home, like forcibly destroying people's crops or deploying troops on the streets, can be carried out in the Andes instead.

A few years earlier, President Reagan had given concrete shape to the notion of a foreign menace by signing a secret National Security Directive which portrayed drugs as a national security threat. By providing cheap, plentiful cocaine to the US, he argued, Andean countries were responsible for poisoning America's youth, undermining the country's social structure and so also its national security. US national security is further threatened by the fact that the Andean countries are themselves at risk of being destabilised by powerful drug traffickers and may go on to 'contaminate' their neighbours. By defining drugs as a national security threat, US intervention abroad can be portrayed as self-defence rather than interference in other countries' internal affairs.

The declaration of 'war' by the US has other important side-effects. One is that, as in other wars, opposition is not easily tolerated. The war takes on the characteristics of a moral crusade: you are either for drugs or against them. Questioning the strategy of the war on drugs means questioning the evil nature of drugs. Those few brave souls in Congress who dare ask if the US anti-drugs strategy is morally right or even workable are shouted down with accusations of being 'soft' on drugs, or 'defeatist'. The fight against drugs is a moral and ideological issue rather than a rational one. For rationally, it defies the most basic laws of free-market capitalism — people supply goods if there's a market for them — whose first champion is the US.

Another side-effect is that with the use of war imagery comes the notion of victory. By calling it a war, people believe it will actually end, in triumph, of course. As Republican congressman Dan Burton put it: 'In war there is no substitute for victory.'[13] In the view of critics, however, drugs are a social problem which, like drunken driving or venereal disease, will never be 'conquered', only managed and, with luck, reduced. By calling it a war, the US is doomed to lose. As victory appears more and more elusive and public disillusionment grows, US policy makers will have two alternatives: to give up, which is unlikely, or to raise the stakes by pouring more and more money, weapons and manpower into the fight. In fact, instead of achieving victory, the drugs war is more likely to result in another Vietnam: 'dirty, inglorious, often futile and seemingly never finished'.[14]

Furthermore, if the war began as simply a figure of speech, it soon turned into the real thing. The war metaphor has created the notion that the way to win is by the power of the gun. It also suggests that 'anything goes', the erosion of civil liberties included, in pursuit of victory. By calling it a war, drugs are to be fought not by scientists, doctors and social workers but by police officers, soldiers and politicians.

Ironically, where other foreign policy and security concerns are considered more important, the fight against drugs is happily relegated to the backburner.

Both the Carter and Reagan administrations turned a blind eye to General Noriega's drug-running activities for years because he was an asset. Although US intelligence sources had linked him to the drug trade since 1972, the Pentagon and the CIA opposed taking action against the Panamanian dictator because of his usefulness as a spy for the CIA and as an ally in US-led efforts to overthrow Nicaragua's Sandinista government. Only in 1986 when his usefulness had expired did these bodies allow an indictment to be brought against Noriega on charges of drug trafficking. In the ultimate of ironies, the 1989 invasion of Panama by US troops, which ousted him, was heralded as a major victory in the 'war on drugs'.

In Central America the US-backed *contras* who tried to overthrow Nicaragua's government in the 1980s were repeatedly accused of involvement in drug trafficking. This was actively encouraged by the CIA in return for help in ousting the Sandinistas. At the same time, with less than conclusive evidence, Washington was extremely vocal in accusing the highest levels of the Sandinista government of active participation in the drugs trade.

At other times, however, the White House has been able usefully to combine the fight against drugs with the fulfilment of other foreign policy objectives, particularly the struggle against radical leftist movements in Latin America. The two goals are combined in the notion of the 'narco-guerrilla' or 'narco-terrorist': in some areas like Peru's Upper Huallaga Valley, the administration maintains that druglords and insurgents work so closely together it is virtually impossible to distinguish between them. In some cases, it argues, it may be necessary to fight insurgents to fight drugs. Critics say this is simply dragging the US down the slippery slope of involvement in one of the world's ugliest insurgencies.

THE differences in views and objectives are hardly surprising considering the labyrinth of agencies involved in the 'war on drugs', each with its own priorities, goals and philosophies. According to one estimate[15] some 58 federal agencies and 74 congressional committees have some part in the drug war. Turf wars, budget battles and bureaucratic in-fighting rage between them, resulting in fragmented and often conflicting policies.

The State Department, for example, is more interested in improving relations with foreign countries than penalising them for not fighting drugs. The Justice Department is geared more towards arresting drug traffickers than using military might to stop them, in contrast to Defense Department personnel who are trained to locate and destroy enemy targets. The Customs Service and Coast Guard regularly squabble over who should get credit for particular drug seizures. In the confused environment of the Andes, inter-agency bickering can be disastrous. 'The various law enforcement agencies,' warned the State Department secretary general in 1990, 'which until now have tended to focus more on internecine disputes over areas of responsibility than on cooperation, will... have to learn how to cooperate abroad.'[16]

In 1988 President Bush set up an Office of National Drug Control Policy to try to coordinate the various agencies and the following year appointed William Bennett as its director. 'I will not tolerate,' Bush lectured his cabinet sternly as he swore Bennett in, 'and the country cannot afford, bureaucratic in-fighting that forces us to fight this battle with one arm tied behind our back.'[17]

A beefy, rumpled figure with rolled-up shirt sleeves, the US's new drugs czar looked more suited to the football pitches of his boyhood than to the dreary bureaucratic machinations of Capitol Hill. With a taste for the bully pulpit and fiery rhetoric, Bennett tackled his job with the same mixture of neo-conservative zeal, impatience and acerbic humour with which he had previously served as minister for education. Described as a 'philosopher by training, a teacher by inclination and a politician mostly by accident',[18] Bennett unquestionably held both the worst and the best job in Washington.

Soon, though, it became clear that it was more 'worst' than 'best'. He was a 'czar without an empire, a general without troops'.[19] To his annoyance, Bennett had been refused a cabinet post and he had no direct authority over the main agencies involved in the fight against drugs like the FBI, the US Customs Service or the DEA. Few in the Justice or State Departments took him seriously. 'They don't pay any attention in the Administration to Bill Bennett' said congressman Charles Rangel in September 1990, one year after Bush had announced his anti-drugs strategy. 'We're in worse shape now than we were before the president's stirring speech a year ago.'[20]

By November, Bennett had 'run out of gas' and handed in his resignation. In March 1991 he was replaced in the $107,300 a year job by former Republican Florida governor and restaurateur, Bob Martinez. Like Bennett, 56-year-old Martinez had a reputation as a hard-line conservative who favoured a law-and-order approach to drugs. But unlike Bennett, he was more of a hands-on man who enjoyed the nitty gritty details of public policy.

WHEN he drew up his $7900-million anti-drug strategy, Bush had four cards to choose from: repression at home; repression abroad; prevention at home (through education or trying to solve the social and economic problems at the root of drug addiction); or prevention abroad (by providing cocaine-producing countries with economic aid which would help lessen the dependence of their economies on cocaine).

Each option had its drawbacks. Repression at home, for example, was the most likely to have an impact on availability of drugs but had the disadvantage that it might trample on civil liberties, which Americans treasure so highly. Compulsory drug testing and unwarranted searches were unlikely to go down well. Prevention at home and abroad was a good idea — many politicians recognised that in the long run it was probably the only solution — but because it was long term not short term there was little political capital to be made out of it. And to work it needed an awful lot of money, more than Congress would ever authorise.

That left repression abroad. This too had its snags. Cocaine-producer countries might not like being made to fight what they saw as America's war. There was a risk that US military advisers sent to supervise operations might get drawn into military conflict. But the option had important advantages: it was far cheaper than 'prevention'; it yielded immediate results, like seizures which could be easily visualised; and it took place so far away from the US that no-one would know or care about abuses of civil liberties.

The anti-drug plan that Bush finally announced in September 1989 was balanced strongly in favour of repression abroad. Around 70 per cent of the budget was allocated to it. The other three options were included too, but their funding was minimal by comparison. At home, for example, prison capacity nearly doubled and stiffer sentences were introduced for users and sellers. More money was also made available for domestic prevention, education and treatment. Abroad, some economic assistance was provided to fund crop substitution and alternative development programmes and drug awareness campaigns.

The international part of Bush's strategy was called the Andean Strategy, a five-year initiative under which the US pledges to give $2,500 million to Bolivia, Peru and Colombia until 1994. The strategy, a mixture of carrot and stick, is divided into three main elements: law enforcement, eradication and economic assistance.

The first strand is law enforcement. This means disrupting traffickers' operations and seizing their assets before cocaine reaches the US. This is done by destroying processing laboratories, seizing planes, tracing and imprisoning the leaders of major trafficking organisations, and blocking shipment of the chemicals used to process cocaine. In theory, when law enforcement is carried out effectively, producers of coca leaf find they have no-one to sell to, the price of coca leaf falls and they turn to other crops.

The second strand is eradication. 'Eradication is elegant, almost beautiful, in its simplicity. Without the wholesale cultivation of the coca plant there is no cocaine trade,' wrote one of Washington's strongest advocates, right winger Andy Messing. 'Simply put, if you don't aerially eradicate you can take the word WIN out of the Cocaine War's vocabulary'.[21] Like Messing, many US officials see eradication of the coca plant as the key to fighting cocaine. They believe that the best way to tackle the drug problem is to go quite literally to its source, the plant itself. In the words of former US ambassador to Bolivia, Edward Corr, 'The closer you get to where it comes from, the more bang you get for your buck.'[22]

Eradication has many attractions. It is much easier to find a coca field in the Andes than a kilo of cocaine on the streets of New York. Coca fields are easily visible from the air. And coca farmers are a lot easier to take on than armed traffickers. Unlike traffickers, farmers cannot afford to prevent detection of their crop or to bribe officials to look the other way.

The cheapest way is to uproot the coca plants by hand. But in Peru the farmers, helped by Maoist rebels and perhaps drug traffickers, fought back. Between 1983 and 1988, 32 Peruvian eradication workers were killed and eradication efforts were suspended for more than a year. Manual eradication was clearly too dangerous, and in any case was unable to keep pace with the new fields of coca which were being planted. Since the early 1980s US scientists had been searching for another method.

In 1987, they found the Magic Bullet solution: a herbicide which could be sprayed from the air, appeared to be environmentally safe, which avoided the need to come into contact with irate coca growers or their guns (if they had them). Its name was Tebuthiuron, commonly known as 'Spike'.

A number of herbicides had been tried before, like 2,4-D, which had been sprayed on Bolivian coca fields in 1982. But of 30 herbicides that had been secretly tested by the US government, Spike was considered by far the most effective. A 1987 report prepared for the State Department declared that Spike destroyed the coca plant while at the same time posing little or no threat to humans or the environment. Spurred on by such assurances, US diplomats in Peru persuaded the government to start tests with Spike.

Environmentalists were not happy. Spike, they said, was an indiscriminate defoliant that could cause irreparable harm to the delicate ecosystem of the Andean jungle. They pointed to the fact that the label warned that Spike 'is an extremely active herbicide which will kill trees, shrubs and other forms of desirable vegetation' and should be 'kept out of lakes, ponds and streams', a difficult proposition on the rain-drenched slopes of the Andes. A report by the US Environmental Protection Agency described Spike as 'mobile to very mobile' in wet soils and warned that if it leached into ground water it could contaminate water supplies. These are some of the reasons why herbicides had been banned in the US for the eradication of marijuana plantations.

In May 1988, plans to use Spike were dealt a mortal blow when its sole manufacturers, Eli Lilly & Company, refused to sell the herbicide to the State Department for coca eradication on the grounds that it might face environmental litigation and retaliation against its employees by drug traffickers. Then came an attack from another direction, from inside the government itself. The US government's chief herbicide scientist, Walter Gentner, resigned, protesting that Spike had not been adequately tested for environmental safety. Andean governments became increasingly uneasy. In 1988 Bolivia passed a law outlawing the use of herbicides. Peru's President Fujimori made it clear that, while he was allowing US scientists to continue tests, he had no intention of ever allowing Spike to be used.

Spike's most passionate supporters were undaunted. 'To win the war on drugs the US must take the war to the coca fields,' declared congressman Dan Burton. The US, he said, must be willing to eradicate South America's coca fields 'with or without the cooperation of its leaders', even though this would be totally illegal. 'If it comes to a choice between offending foreign leaders by violating their borders to kill coca plants and seeing hundreds of thousands of young Americans die or be ruined for life because cocaine is so readily available on our streets, there is no choice to be made.'[23] Inside the State Department, however, officials were having a change of heart. Given the social and political consequences of eradication, they realised the only way they could persuade farmers to accept eradication was to make it voluntary, in exchange for compensation.

Scientists at the US Agriculture Department, meanwhile, are still continuing the secret search for another chemical or biological 'quick fix' to destroy coca at the source.[24] In early 1990 the administration more than quadrupled the Department's budget to $6.5 million.

One of their most bizarre ideas, nicknamed the 'bugs for drugs' proposal, was to unleash swarms of a tiny white coca-eating moth, known as the malumbia, into the jungles of South America. The insect would be bred in mass quantities at home then air-dropped into coca regions as eggs or caterpillars. In March 1990, Wlademar Klassen, associate deputy administrator for the Agricultural Research Service which oversees the project, declared 'it looks promising'.[25] Other scientists and environmentalists were less optimistic. 'How do you keep it from eating legitimate crops? What would make this moth stay within its political boundaries?' asked Walt Gentner, the scientist who had resigned over Spike. Environmentalists feared use of the moth would simply drive coca farmers to douse their coca crops with huge quantities of insecticides to kill the pests.[26]

In 1990, the US government's scientific research labs came up with another idea: to engineer coca leaves genetically so that they no longer produce cocaine. Under the proposal, which has been shown to officials of the Office of National Drug Control Policy, the CIA, the FBI and the DEA, an altered gene whose product blocks one of the enzymes that makes cocaine would be transmitted via a plant virus to attack coca plants world-wide. 'Given the choice of adversaries, I'd rather wage a campaign against a vegetable than slug it out with the Medellín cartel,' said Boston physicist Russell Seitz, a leading advocate of the proposal. Plant virologist Roger Beachy of Washington University in St Louis, however, called it 'biological warfare of the worst kind'.

The third main strand of anti-drugs strategy is economic aid. Under the Bush plan, crop substitution and other economic revival programmes are to be carried out once law enforcement has, in theory, made countries safe and coca fields have been destroyed. Whereas the Andean countries, which see cocaine as an economic problem, view economic aid as a precondition to wiping out cocaine, Washington sees it as a reward for cooperation. This is partly because many US officials are repelled by the notion of paying a country to stop producing something illegal. According to congressional researcher, Rafael Perl, some see it as comparable to paying nations to stop hijacking aircraft or taking hostages.[27] The first year of the plan provided little economic assistance, and conditioned future aid on Andean countries meeting eradication and interdiction (drug and lab seizures) targets and carrying out US-approved economic policies, a strategy a 1990 US Committee on Government Operations report found 'unworkable and unreasonable'.[28]

The amount of economic aid promised by the US under the Andean Strategy, although higher than ever before, is insignificant when set against the revenues earned by the drugs industry. In 1991, for example, Bolivia was authorised $98.5 million in US economic aid. It sounds a lot, until you bear in mind that cocaine brings between $300 and $600 million a year into the Bolivian economy.

Another important element of US drugs strategy is certification. To ensure the Andean countries fight the war against cocaine in accordance with US guidelines, like eradication and seizure targets, every year the US president has to 'certify' that drug-producing nations are cooperating with the US in fighting drugs or are taking adequate steps on their own. Each country receives a sort of end-of-year report which says 'is improving' or 'could do better'. Countries that fail the test may be punished by having part of their aid suspended or by having trade sanctions imposed against them.

Recently the procedure has come under attack both from the Andean nations, who see it as humiliating, and from Congressmen who complain that it is a dog with no bite. This is because Bush, and Reagan before him, have never used their powers to punish a close ally. Year after year they have given the green light to all major drug-producing countries, regardless of how well they have done, arguing that punitive measures would damage relations between these countries and the US and make them less, not more, cooperative in the future. The only countries US presidents have been willing to decertify are countries with which the US has no relations anyway, like Afghanistan, Iran, Syria (at least until recently) and Myanmar (Burma).

US strategy also places considerable emphasis on extradition of major traffickers to the US, a subject which has long been a bugbear in relations with Andean countries. Washington says it is necessary because their judicial systems have become so corrupted by drugs that they no longer function effectively. In Colombia, for example, judges face a choice between *plata* and *plomo*, between accepting bribes from the traffickers, or a bullet in the head. But South Americans see extradition as an attack on their sovereignty and a measure which is politically unacceptable at home. In any case, they argue, there is little long-term point in extradition since when you extradite one druglord, there are always ten more to fill his shoes. As the Spanish proverb goes, *a rey muerto, rey puesto* (literally: for every dead king you have a new king).

SLOWLY but surely, the war that started as a metaphor has turned into the real thing. Seeing all previous tactics fail, Washington looked to guns, soldiers and strong-arm tactics for a solution.

The turning point came on 18 September 1989, when Defense Secretary Richard Cheney announced that the Pentagon would be given the lead role in detecting and monitoring the entry of drugs into the US by air or sea. Abroad, the military's mission would be to control borders, carry out aerial and maritime surveillance and train Andean troops. US Special Forces personnel in the field would be stepped up. The Pentagon was also ordered to centralise drugs intelligence information into a single communications network.

The Pentagon's agreement, however, came only after years of soul-searching. Many US military were (and still are) vehemently opposed to the idea of getting dragged into a war which was clearly unwinnable and for which they would become the scapegoat. The role of the military, they argued, was to defend the US against attacks by foreign nations, not drug smugglers. In 1988, Caspar Weinberger, Cheney's predecessor, warned that 'calling for the use of the government's full military resources to put a stop to the drug trade makes for hot and exciting rhetoric. But responding to those calls... would make for terrible national security policy, poor politics and guaranteed failure in the campaign against drugs.'[29]

Opponents of involvement of the US military believed it threatened the precedent established in the Posse Comitatus Act of 1878, more than 100 years earlier. The law, passed immediately after the Civil War in which federal troops had occupied the defeated South, forbade the use of the military in civil law enforcement activities.

Then, in April 1986, Reagan signed his National Security Directive, which declared drugs a matter of national security and gave authority to the military to plan assaults, equip police forces and to transport them to sites of action. If the main function of the military was to neutralise serious external threats to national security, now drugs posed such a threat. 'Our soldiers, sailors and airmen are being paid to protect the national security,' wrote conservative columnist James Kilpatrick.[30] 'Let them earn their pay.' Three months later 160 US troops and six US Air Force Black Hawk helicopters were sent to Bolivia to take part in a major drugs bust called Operation Blast Furnace.

In 1988 a bill called the Omnibus Anti Drug Abuse Act increased military aid to countries involved in US anti-drugs programmes and waived a 1974 ban on aid to foreign police, introduced because of human rights abuses. The act also gave the US military powers of search, seizure and arrest outside the US.

By the time Cheney gave the Pentagon the lead role in the fight against drugs in 1989, another factor had entered the equation: the thaw in relations between the super powers. With the end of the cold war, the Pentagon lacked a mission and risked having its budget and manpower slashed. The war on drugs could solve both problems and provide valuable jungle warfare training too. As Major Susan Flores stated in the *Marine Corps Gazette*, 'In a time when there will be increasing demands for fiscal constraints and selective spending, Congress has already demonstrated that it is willing to provide funding for counter-narcotics programs. Before the Marine Corps says "No" to drugs, it should think seriously about what is to be gained.' Outright opposition to military involvement in the drugs war was replaced by emphasis on increased funding as a condition for involvement.

Administration officials justified the military build-up in the Andes by saying that troops and weaponry were a rational response to the growing ruthlessness and sophistication of the drug traffickers which were over-powering police and DEA agents. Bennett used increasingly lurid terms to deplore the 'bad guys'. 'The traffickers view violence, threats and murder as tools of their dirty trade,' he warned in June 1990. Melvyn Levitsky claimed: 'We are simply reacting to reality.'[31]

Once the Pentagon was involved, it seemed logical to involve Andean military forces with whom it already had close links and could talk to as 'man to man'. Despite having some of the worst human rights records in the world, Andean armies were co-opted into the drugs war. Law enforcement assistance that had previously been given to Andean police forces was switched to military aid. Military aid to the Andes leapt from $22 million in the fiscal year 1989 to an unprecedented $131 million in the fiscal year 1990 and to $151 million in 1991. By 1991 the region had outstripped Central America to become the largest recipient of US military aid in Latin America.

In December 1989 US troops invaded Panama. For the first time, the US showed it was willing to wage real wars to tackle cocaine.

ON 6 September 1990, Bennett blew out the candles on a cake to celebrate the first birthday of his drugs strategy. Addressing a Senate hearing, he was buoyant. The price of cocaine was rising in some US cities and purity was down, two sure indicators that law enforcement operations had hit the traffickers' supplies. In the last quarter of 1989 and first half of 1990 cocaine-related deaths and medical emergencies had plunged and the number of high school and college students using cocaine had dropped by nearly half. Abroad, several traffickers had been extradited to the US and a record number of processing laboratories had been destroyed.

Despite the media razzmatazz, however, lay (and lies) a more sombre picture. The number of drugs-provoked murders, for example, had soared. In Washington DC, which Bennett had promised to turn into a test case for his drugs-control policies, murders reached record levels in 1990 and again in 1991. Although casual cocaine use had fallen, hard-core abuse and addiction were still rising. Many experts feared too that declining cocaine purity and rising prices might not mean, as Bennett hoped, a slackening in demand or supply, but might merely be temporary fluctuations of a moving market or the results of market manipulation by traffickers. The druglords might be trying to compensate for profits lost to seizures or capitalising on consumers' fears of a cocaine shortage. Declining purity could be a deliberate ploy to boost their profits.

In Washington DC, residents' fears that the drugs problem was out of control had heightened when their mayor, Marion Barry, had been arrested in January 1990 and charged with possessing crack. Barry, who had promised to turn the city into a 'drug-free zone', had walked into an FBI undercover operation in a hotel on the city's shadowy 14th Street and been videotaped handing dollars to a woman in exchange for drugs.

Abroad, although seizures were up, production was rocketing even faster. By March 1990, Latin America was churning out an estimated 775 metric tonnes of cocaine a year, nearly twice the amount of a few years earlier. Coca fields were expanding by around 10 per cent a year. Seizures, although up, still represented less than 1 per cent of cocaine produced. In fact, it made little difference how much the enforcement agents seized since South America produces enough cocaine to meet world demand several times over. US demand alone could be met with a mere 14 per cent of the world coca crop. Just as depressing was the fact that even if anti-drugs agents did dent Andean production, there was no guarantee this would affect the street price in Miami or New York. According to research by Peter Reuter of the RAND Corporation, if the cocaine supply was miraculously reduced by 50 per cent, this would raise the street price in the US only 4 per cent a kilo. In fact, the price would probably not rise at all because traffickers and US dealers, who make the biggest markups, might decide to bear the losses themselves.

Western experts were also painfully helpless when it came to controlling conditions in the Andean countries where cocaine is grown and manufactured. People in those countries seemed to have far more reasons for growing coca than for destroying it. There was one country, in particular, which appeared to be incurably addicted and was threatening to become one of the world's largest cocaine producers. That was Bolivia.

2

Snowfields:
The Farmers

Sinahota

> *I'm off to Sinahota, a shabby little town*
>
> *Where they sell* pichicata *to make the country fall apart*
>
> *I'm off in my old banger to a cardboard town*
>
> *Of* narcos *from Sacata, Otros and El Bolson*
>
> *I grow my little coca bushes and stomp them on the road*
>
> *So that* narcos *and little soldiers can stuff their wallets*
>
> *They call me a* zepe *as I carry bundles of coca leaves*
>
> *And* pichicata *for junkies and* señores
>
> *At the far end of Sinahota where the vultures perch*
>
> *They sell* pichicata *like sweets, like sweets*

Bolivian pop song

THE TOWN's real name is Sinahota, but the locals call it Little Chicago because it is in the heart of Bolivia's Chapare region, where most of the country's coca leaf (the raw material for cocaine) is grown. As in Chicago, violence is never far below the surface as druglords in denim jackets settle scores with regular shootouts. At first sight, though, Sinahota's sprawl of corrugated iron-roofed shacks looks like any other town on the Cochabamba to Santa Cruz highway. Bowler-hatted Indian women sell locally grown mandarins and contraband Reebok shoes at street-side stalls. *Compro dólares*, reads a sign strung over one. There is even a *Salón de Belleza Unisex*. Only the carcasses of Studebakers and Chevrolets which rust by the roadside, the seedy dance and billiards halls and myriad hotels give a glimpse of the cocaine wealth which the town wears like a moth-eaten fur coat over its clothes of rags.

Apart from the passing lorries on the main road, it is quiet here by day. Young men drink Paceña beer in its bars while they wait for something to happen. Others sleep away the midday heat in the wooden cages above, like rabbit hutches, which serve as living quarters. Beside the town's food market, tiny bedraggled children in oversized T-shirts splash barefoot in the puddles left by a tropical deluge as *salsa* music blasts from a shack opposite. In the prefab which serves as the Town Hall, the mayor, Juan Carlos Segovia, attends to the problems of his flock, like the schoolteacher who has run out of classrooms. 'We have 1,000 pupils,' he groans, 'but we've only got room for 300. We're now having to teach the middle school kids in private houses. We'd like to build a new school, but where will the money come from?' The only thing that cheers him up is that Sinahota is about to get electricity. 'We hope to open a Kivon ice-cream parlour,' Segovia says excitedly. On the wall behind is a photograph of his inauguration as mayor. Around his neck he wears a garland of coca leaves, the only thing that ever brought the town luck.

At the far end of town, out of sight of the main road and just before the shacks merge into jungle and coca fields, is a huge hangar packed with *campesinos* who hook bulging sacks onto weighing scales. By day this is the hub of the town's activity: the *Venta de Coca* or Coca Market. The pungent spinach-like smell of the green leaves pervades the air. Their price is a barometer of the cocaine trade: if the cocaine dealers have avoided the cops, demand is strong and prices high. When there has been a raid, prices slump. Today business is brisk: a 100-pound bundle, called a *carga*, is selling at around 250 *bolivianos* ($80), compared to 200 ($60) the week before.

Many of the sacks are unloaded from big trucks which belong to middlemen who have bought the leaves from coca farmers and hope to sell them at a profit at the market. Other *cocaleros* (coca growers) bring their own. As they enter the market each pays one *boliviano* (30 cents), a sort of 'coca tax' collected by the Town Hall. Who buys the leaves is more difficult to say, and it is better not to ask. In theory, the buyers are wholesalers who sell them to peasants who chew them, as their ancestors have for centuries, to stave off hunger and fatigue. In reality, everybody knows that virtually all the leaves will be bought by drug mafia middlemen and mashed with chemicals at secret jungle laboratories to produce Bolivia's Number One export: cocaine.

The leaves reach the labs on the backs of carriers known as *zepes*, or ants. They carry several sack loads at a time along jungle trails, usually by night to avoid the police. Over the years the police have learnt the trails, and often stand in waiting for the *zepes* just outside town. Like the mayor they levy a tax, but since the transport of leaves for processing into cocaine is illegal they can charge much higher rates, around $3 a time.

It is at night that Sinahota springs to life. Young men who have been resting at home or in one of the town's scores of cheap hotels during the day spill into the streets, secure under the cloak of darkness. Their business is *pichicata* or *la merca* (the merchandise), the words locals use for cocaine. A few buy it to get high; others, the *pichicateros*, buy it to process further into finished cocaine. It is a dangerous time to wander about if you are not doing 'business'. Many of the traffickers consume their products and can behave unpredictably. Often there are Mafia-style shootouts between *pichicateros*.

Sinahota is also where the traffickers buy 'precursor' chemicals, particularly kerosene (paraffin), needed to process coca leaves into cocaine. They are sold by Juanita who owns the petrol station at the far end of town. She has a licence to sell petrol for cars and kerosene for cooking but siphons off a portion to sell to traffickers at a markup. She sells kerosene, for example, at 150 *bolivianos* ($45) a 10-litre barrel when it is legal, 200 *bolivianos* ($60) if for cocaine. By day, when business is sluggish, she embroiders cushion covers and minds her children. Serious trading begins at midnight.

After a night's work the *pichicateros* relax over a beer. On Saturdays they let off steam in one of the open-air dance halls, like the *Lucero* (Morning Star), which looks like the coca market hangar except that it has psychedelic paintings on the far wall and tables and chairs for the guests. Sometimes the traffickers bump into Bolivian anti-drugs police, known as Leopards, or American DEA agents in civvies from their base at Chimoré, 20 minutes' drive east. But since everybody is off duty nobody pays much attention and gets on with having a good time.

The cocaine trade in Sinahota today, however, is a shadow of what it used to be. In the early 1980s, when consumers in the West began to clamour for cocaine, there was so much dope in Sinahota that a pop group from Cochabamba wrote a song about it. Coca paste, the clay-coloured powder produced in the first stage of processing the leaf into cocaine, was sold alongside mandarins and rice as if it were flour. 'On one side of the street were the plastic bags of dope. On the other were rows of weighing scales where the buyers weighed it to check they weren't being cheated,' recalls Jorge, a Sinahota resident who today is queueing to see the mayor. Also on sale were do-it-yourself kits to enable locals to set up their own paste-making pits in jungle clearings near their homes.

Every trail from Sinahota into the forest led to these pits, and law and order was so lax that people barely bothered to hide them. You could even see some from the main road. The crystalline River Chapare turned red with chemicals poured into it by *campesinos* after they had used them for processing.

'The cocaine paste was then flown out of the Chapare region by small planes which used an airstrip built by Gulf Oil just outside Sinahota,' says Jorge. 'They flew it to big labs east of here, near Santa Cruz, where it was turned into cocaine. You could hear the drone of small planes all day long. The authorities didn't interfere because the traffickers and even the *campesinos* were well armed and killed anyone that tried to come near. The town was a free zone.'

Dripping with gold chains and rings, the druglords swaggered through town like Miami gangsters. They were the old breed of trafficker who bragged about their vast wealth and threw wild and raucous parties: they had not yet been forced to learn that the best way to do business is to keep a low profile. One establishment, the *Restaurante Oriente*, had to replace its roof three times because one druglord had the inconvenient habit of proving his *machismo* by shooting at the ceiling.

The price of the coca leaf rocketed and no-one could get into the business fast enough. One resident, Carmen Fernández, remembers the day in 1984 when a *carga* fetched the all-time high of $800.

The price was already around $600. Then one night the word spread that it had hit $800. Everybody rushed to the coca market, scraping up every leaf they could find. Because of the rush to sell the price immediately fell to $400. I was unlucky because my coca plants weren't ready for harvesting that day. When I took some leaves the following week the price was back down at $250 a *carga*.

From a marginal jungle village, Sinahota swelled into a town of 10,000 inhabitants. Because there were not enough houses to accommodate them, many squatted in tents. On Sundays the town held fairs, attended by 4,000 to 5,000 people who bartered cocaine for food mixers and hair dryers. It was Sinahota's heyday.

Hotel owners and *restaurateurs* made a killing, catering for the hordes of strangers, usually Colombians or Brazilians, who passed through town 'on business'. Their residences are still the best in town today. Others fronted their money by building dance halls like the *Lucero* and the *Padrino* (Godfather) where they invited well known groups to play.

Professions without links to the cocaine trade began to feel the pinch. Teachers, like the mayor, quit their classrooms, realising they could make over ten times more growing coca. 'I was earning $30 a month,' he recalls. 'Growing coca I could earn up to $400 a month. We all planted up.' Farmers uprooted their rice or bananas and replaced them with coca seedlings. Soon coca was virtually the only thing people knew how to grow.

Inebriated with their fairytale wealth, Sinahota's inhabitants squandered their money on status symbols like Datsun trucks or Toyota land cruisers, which traffickers smuggled from countries like Brazil as a way of recycling their cocaine dollars. They sold at ridiculously low prices. You could buy a Volkswagen Beetle from Brazil, for example, for as little as $300, provided you paid cash. Others bought leather jackets, gold chains and ghetto blasters, or simply better food for the family. 'We lived well then,' remembers Carmen. 'We ate meat most days and we bought medicines for the children when they got ill.'

The favourite way of spending the new wealth was to drink. Villagers ordered beer or whisky by the crate or by the square metre, forming habits which later they would be unable to kick. 'Everyone drank, it was virtually the only thing they could think of doing with their money,' says Carmen. 'The attitude was "Enjoy today, for tomorrow you may die".'

Some made half-hearted attempts to put by some of their money in the bank at the nearby village of Villa Tunari, half an hour along the main road to Cochabamba, or buried piles of *peso* notes (as the currency was then) in the ground. Most, though, could not see the point since inflation was running at several thousand per cent a year and money was worthless as soon as you got it. The best way to invest it was to spend it. In any case, even if they had wanted to save, few knew how.

The drawback was that other prices shot up too. The cost of living soared from $20 to $100 a day, making Sinahota one of the most expensive towns in Bolivia. Products also used to manufacture cocaine, like toilet paper and kerosene, became so expensive and scarce that few could afford to buy them. Still today toilet rolls, if you can find them, cost the equivalent of 30 US cents each, around double what they cost elsewhere. Now that farmers had torn up their food crops, food was far more expensive because it had to be imported by truck from the nearest city, six hours' drive away, Cochabamba.

In August 1984 the bubble burst. Realising the Chapare had fallen outside government control, President Hernán Siles Zuazo sent in the army and police. They occupied the area for the next six months and destroyed hundreds of cocaine paste-making set-ups, some of them with as many as 140 maceration pits. There was even a lab inside an abandoned bus.

The price of coca leaf plummeted. By September 1984 it had fallen to $500 a *carga*, and the following year continued to tumble. The population of Sinahota dwindled too, falling from 10,000 to its present level of around 1,000.

The cocaine traffickers, hounded by the police, moved their operations deeper into the jungle to an area north of Sinahota which the locals call the *Zona Roja* (Red Zone) or Cocaine Alley. This centres around the dirt roads that branch off the Cochabamba to Santa Cruz highway just before Sinahota. Isinuta, a village about an hour's drive north off the main road, took over Sinahota's banner of notoriety. In the rainy season parts of the road are flooded by rivers and only four-wheel drive vehicles can make the journey. But for the traffickers the town's inaccessibility is its greatest virtue.

Today Sinahota has little to show for its boom years. Living conditions remain as squalid as ever: the streets are still unpaved, turning into rivers of mud when the summer rains come, the houses stay unlit (except those of people rich enough to afford a private generator). The children of Sinahota, like children in Bolivia as a whole, have the highest mortality rate in South America. Three in 20 die before they reach the age of five. At least one in ten children under five is seriously malnourished.[1]

'Drugs haven't helped us. Rather, they have undermined our reputation. If you come from Sinahota people assume you are a druggie,' says the mayor. Sinahota is tired of living with the Leopards and DEA agents. 'The Leopards maltreat us even though we're not guilty. Two or three years ago they used to steal everything in the town, cars, motorbikes, anything they fancied. They even stole the kids' school-books. They have got better now, mainly because there's nothing here now for them to seize.' But finding work outside the cocaine industry is still extremely difficult. 'People can't grow anything else because there's no market,' says the mayor. 'I grew tomatoes, for example, but they earned so little I might as well have given them away.'

IMAGINE there existed a crop that yielded up to four or five harvests a year, for which there was a seemingly limitless demand, and which earned the farmer more than any other product. Imagine there existed a crop that needed hardly any pesticides, that flourished in acidic rain-washed soils in which other crops withered and died, and that was highly labour intensive, providing employment and income for hundreds of impoverished *campesinos* and foreign exchange for the nation. Imagine too, that instead of having to travel hundreds of miles along pot-holed dirt roads to take the crop to market, the farmer simply had to dump it outside his door and wait for it to be picked up.

Such a crop exists. It is an attractive shrub which grows chest high and yields hundreds of green leaves, about two inches long which look like flimsy bay leaves. When it flowers, it produces a delicate white blossom. It is called coca.

Were it not considered illicit by the international community, coca might be the ideal crop for a developing country like Bolivia, which has plentiful supplies of cheap labour and since independence from Spain in 1828 has relied on exporting primary commodities to the developed world for its survival.

One of coca's greatest advantages is that it produces up to five harvests a year, providing the *campesino* with a regular cash flow, which he sees as the equivalent to going to the bank. Most other cash crops, by contrast, produce only one or two harvests a year so that for much of the year the farmer has no income. Frequent harvesting also means labour can be spread over the year, unlike for other crops which need it only once or twice. The leaves can be harvested before the bush is a year old, in contrast with most other cash crops, which take several years to produce their first harvest.

Coca's greatest advantage, though, is that it can be turned into a substance which fuels a multibillion dollar industry and for which there is a seemingly inexhaustible demand. Since that demand took off in the early 1980s, hundreds of thousands of Bolivian peasants have abandoned their homes, wives and pigs in the cold Andean Altiplano (highland plateau) and descended, as gold miners had done before, into the lowlands where coca grows best. Because most coca is illicit, nobody knows for sure how much is grown. Estimates vary from 51,000 to 90,000 hectares, the lower figure being that given by the DEA.

The country's largest coca-growing area is the Chapare, a superbly beautiful region of subtropical rain forests, vermilion sunsets and vast rushing rivers, located half way between the snow-capped Andean mountains and the steamy lowlands of the Amazon basin in the east. The region, a little bigger than Wales, produces around 90 per cent of Bolivia's coca leaf and almost all is for cocaine. In 1990 between 35,230 and 51,198 hectares were estimated to be planted with coca in the Chapare.[2] Bolivian law defines the area as a 'transitional' zone, which means that from 1992 coca cultivation will be illegal and must be phased out by that date. Until 1992 farmers are given $2,000 compensation for every hectare they destroy. After that their coca crops will, theoretically at least, be destroyed by force.

Apart from its climate, the Chapare's relative inaccessibility makes it an ideal centre for the cultivation of coca and the production of cocaine. Although the region is served with a road, funded by the US Agency for International Development (USAID) in 1971 as part of a deliberate effort by the government to colonise the region and take the pressure off the highlands, in the rainy season the stretch from the city of Cochabamba to the Chapare's main town, Villa Tunari, can be cut off for days at a time. Even in the dry season, the road is so full of pot-holes that the six-hour drive from Cochabamba by bus or truck is an endurance test only made tolerable by views of the magnificent mist-veiled mountains which tower on either side.

As they enter the Chapare vehicles are stopped and searched for drugs or 'precursor' chemicals used to process them. At the checkpoints children sell fried fish and trays of red jellies, while anti-drugs police mount the buses and force the drowsy passengers to open their cloth bundles. When the passengers are Indian women, the police frisk their multi-layered silky skirts, which provide a well known hiding place for money and drugs.

The first checkpoint is at Villa Tunari, half an hour before Sinahota. Until the cocaine boom, wealthy residents of Cochabamba used to spend weekends here. They built themselves Italian-style villas with swimming pools and gardens of hibiscus or stayed in the town's hotels with fancy names like Las Vegas and Las Palmas. But the traffickers, who arrived in the early 1980s, scared the *cochabambinos* away. Their houses fell into ruins and the swimming pools turned green and filled with croaking frogs. A few doors down the road from Las Vegas, the offices of the coca eradication agency, DIRECO, were the scene of a bloody confrontation one June day in 1988 between demonstrating coca farmers and the narcotics police. The peasants had come to protest against reports that their fields were to be sprayed with herbicides. As the farmers approached the DIRECO offices, the police apparently panicked and fired their automatic rifles. By sunset 13 peasants were dead, some of them after drowning as they tried to escape by swimming across torrential rivers.

Hotels like Las Palmas and Las Vegas attracted a new kind of customer: first, in the early 1980s, drug traffickers; then, as the US leaned on the Bolivian government to do something about cocaine, development workers. The workers' favourite hangout after a sweaty day's work in the jungle is Las Palmas, a friendly roadside motel famous for its *surubí*, a succulent white fish with a chicken-like texture which thrives in the Chapare rivers.

Bolivia's other main coca growing area is the Yungas, an equally remote region of warm valleys northeast of the capital La Paz. The drive here entails winding four hours along a terrible road which clings tenuously to the edge of jungle-covered mountains which, just a few yards from the road, plunge into 1,000-foot ravines. Scores of makeshift wooden crosses beside the route testify to the drivers who took the bends too quickly or did not bother to mend their brakes before doing the journey.

Because of the Yungas' steep terrain, coca is grown on terraces. In contrast to the Chapare, coca has been grown here for over 2,000 years, used by the peasants for chewing, or *acullicu*, as they laboured in the fields. Smaller and sweeter than the acidic Chapare coca leaf, much of the Yungas leaf is still used today for legal home consumption. For this purpose, 12,000 hectares of coca in the Yungas are defined as legal. Coca grown outside this delineated area, or coca grown to make cocaine, is illegal. Because traffickers pay far better prices than legal leaf merchants, some Yungas leaf is undoubtedly being used to make cocaine. In 1990 an estimated 14,100 hectares of coca were planted in the Yungas,[3] around half of which was probably used to make cocaine.

As the authorities have clamped down on the Chapare and Yungas, coca farmers are now pushing deeper into virgin jungle to avoid detection. This has led to a new area of cultivation in remote areas like the Isiboro Securé

National Park in the northern Chapare. By law coca growing in this area is illegal and subject to forcible eradication without compensation.

Overall, the area of coca continues to grow. Even when eradication campaigns manage to cut the number of hectares planted with coca by several thousand, even more are planted with new coca. In 1989 coca cultivation rose around 9 per cent, according to the US State Department. Cutting back coca is like trying to cut the heads of the hydra in Greek mythology: the more you cut it, the more it grows back. Cut it in one place, it simply pops up in another.

MIGUEL Paredes, aged 55, lives with his wife, Rosana, and his four children in Entre Ríos (Between Rivers), a hamlet about half an hour's drive up a dirt track which branches off the main road near Sinahota. His one-roomed wooden plank house perches on stilts to protect it from snakes and heavy rains. There is little inside: a couple of bamboo beds, some grubby clothes hanging from nails in the wooden beams, a small wood-fire cooking stove and some aluminium pots. There is no electricity, and water has to be collected from the river one kilometre away.

Outside, chickens and children peck about beneath the house. On the scorched earth in front is a pale green carpet of coca leaves, which have turned brittle and pale in the midday sun. Paredes, one of around 300,000 Chapare farmers and their families who depend on coca for a living, is making the most of a spell of dry weather. If the leaves get wet, they go black and rotten and become worthless. Once he had to throw a harvest away.

His face is protected from the sun by a wide-brimmed straw hat. Paredes also wears an ancient Adidas track-suit jacket and baggy black pants supported at the waist with a piece of string. On his feet he wears black rubber sandals made out of old bicycle tyres. His teeth are stained brown by years of coca chewing. Apart from his two hectares of coca, Paredes grows bananas and mandarins. The trees help provide shade for the coca and an insurance against a fall in price of the coca leaf.

Like many *cocaleros*, or coca farmers, Paredes does not come from the Chapare. He is from the village of Tolapalca, in the Altiplano near Oruro, Bolivia's largest mining city. He used to scratch a living from the barren highland earth by raising pigs and sheep, and growing maize. Then, in 1983, a catastrophic drought struck and the animals began to die off one by one. Within a couple of months they had been reduced to a pile of stinking corpses which Paredes could not even bury because the ground was so hard. The maize was so parched he had to throw it away.

'I had literally nothing. There was nothing for it but to move elsewhere,' recalls Paredes, looking towards the forested mountains as if to spot his highland village. 'I suggested the idea to my wife, but she didn't want to leave her mother and the rest of her family; people in the highlands are shy, you know, they don't like change. So I went on my own.

'At first it was hard getting used to the hot climate. In the evening the mosquitoes ate me alive and stopped me sleeping. Many of my friends developed chest complaints. Some went back home, one even died, but most struggled on and tried to get used to it.'

He pauses to stuff a handful of fresh coca leaves into his mouth from a plastic bag he keeps in his pocket.

Finding a plot of land wasn't easy because the Chapare was already very full; people had been flooding in from the Altiplano over the years. I found one plot in an area called Carrasco but it was poor quality and often got flooded so the crops were destroyed. Next I found a place down the road from here, but you could only get to it by crossing several rivers by canoe. Often our provisions and our clothes fell into the water on the way. I had to go to La Paz to sort out the papers giving the land titles. That was very expensive: I had to pay the bus fare and, on top, bribes to the right people.

Finally I managed to get these five hectares here in Entre Ríos where my family joined me. I tried to plant coca because prices were very high. But people were jealous of their coca and it was virtually impossible to get hold of seeds or seedlings. Instead you had to work 15 to 30 days for someone who owned a coca plot, then at the end they'd give you some seeds. But the guy I worked for was a swindler and never paid me, so one night I stole some seeds.

I planted them into special seed-beds, which we call *almácigos*, then a few weeks later planted the seedlings out into the field, shading them with banana trees. After six or eight months they were already producing good sized leaves and at 18 months were giving a proper harvest.

In 1985 there was another influx of people into the Chapare. Many were miners from barren highland cities like Oruro and Potosí who had lost their jobs when the tin price collapsed. Reduced to one meal a day of bread and potatoes, around 5,000 decided to use their indemnification payments to migrate to the Chapare. Now that one boom-bust commodity had bust, they were ready to try another. They settled in colonies like the one in Chimoré, still called *Los Mineros*, and planted coca as fast as they could, slashing and burning the rain forests as they went.

Others were driven to the Chapare by the worst economic crisis in Bolivia's history. Between 1980 and 1985 the gross national product dropped 20 per cent and official unemployment more than tripled from 6 to 20 per cent. In 1985 hyper-inflation had spiralled to a dizzy-making 24,000 per cent a year, the highest level recorded anywhere in the world since the Second World War. Watching the *peso* (the currency that preceded the *boliviano*) was like watching a fruit machine running out of control: zeros kept being added at an uncontrollable speed. As people watched their savings disappear overnight, coca was the only safety valve.

Paredes harvests his coca fields four times a year, gathering the leaves into a cotton sack he wears across his shoulder. When he can afford it he takes on a couple of labourers, usually lads from the Altiplano looking for seasonal jobs. He pays them eight *bolivianos* ($2.5) a day, but on top has to feed them, give them coca to chew and somewhere to sleep. The leaves are spread out to dry to draw out the cocaine alkaloids and make them lose two-thirds of their weight, then stuffed into nylon sacks to make 100-pound bundles, or *cargas*. Paredes takes them to market in Sinahota, or spreads the word that he has some coca to sell and waits for someone to pick it up at the door of his home. Often the buyers are neighbours, but he never asks them what will be done with the leaves. He just sells to who pays most.

Because the price of coca continually fluctuates, Paredes's income does too. In January 1990, for example, the price dropped to an all-time low of $10 a *carga*, but later in the year sold at ten times that. By March 1991 it was about $70. On average Paredes earns between $1,000 and $2,500 a year per hectare, around a tenth of what he would have earned ten years ago. From this he deducts about $30 for production costs (workers' wages, fertilisers and so on) which leaves a final income from the two hectares of about $4,000. Given Bolivia's average per capita income of $570, that means big bucks, although Paredes says his family still struggles to survive. The two eldest children are at school so need books. If one gets ill he has to buy medicines: Bolivia's are the most expensive in the world.

Paredes also knows that what he earns for his coca leaves is a fraction of their final value when sold on the streets of New York as cocaine. His two hectares will eventually be turned into 18 kilograms of pure cocaine worth between $360,000 and $720,000. Paredes thus earns around 0.5 per cent of his coca crop's final value. 'It's like any commodity,' he reflects, 'the poor get the bum deal. The people that make the big money don't live in Bolivia but in America.'

AS MORE and more *Chapareños* rushed to grow coca leaf in the early 1980s, driving prices down, growing numbers decided to increase their profits by carrying out the next stage of the cocaine manufacturing process, the making of paste. Many were reluctant at first, and some still are: if they made paste they could no longer claim that they were growing a traditional crop that had nothing to do with the cocaine industry. Paste was, plain and simple, illegal. Running paste pits also went against the way of thinking of many *campesinos* who were used to subsisting on the land, not being entrepreneurs. Some could not find the necessary $100 or so capital to set up a pit.

Many soon overcame their doubts as they realised the considerable benefits: a hectare of coca leaf worth, say, $2,400, turned into cocaine paste worth almost double. By 1985 police estimated there were around 5,000 pits in the Chapare, one for every eight coca-growing families. Sometimes they were communal pits run by farmers who pooled their resources. More often they were run by small-time traffickers who were employed by the big guys or worked freelance, selling it to whoever paid best.

The drug barons were delighted. Before, they had made paste themselves in secret labs in the Beni, an hour's flight by small plane north of the Chapare. With peasants making the paste in the same area as they grew the leaf, this cut out the risks involved in transporting the leaf to the labs. *Campesinos* took the risk instead. The *narcos* only had to transport the less bulky and more valuable paste and could concentrate on the next, much more profitable, stages in the process, the manufacture of cocaine base and hydrochloride (finished cocaine).

Gradually, as more and more *campesinos* made paste and the price fell, people were forced to move further up the ladder to keep up their incomes and made base as well, often in the same laboratory. Again, the druglords were delighted.

Anyone can make a pit or *pozo*. A hole is dug in the ground, usually beside a river because water is needed for the processing, and lined with plastic sheeting pegged down in the four corners with sticks. If there is a risk of rain, more plastic sheeting is hung over the pit for protection.

Making paste is as easy as cooking apple pie. People know the recipe so well, they do not need to write it down. If they did it might read as follows:

Cocaine Paste

To make 1 kg you need:

> 96 kg coca leaf
> 1 litre sulphuric acid
> 11 litres kerosene (paraffin)
> 4 kg lime

The process is masterminded by a chemist whom they call the *cocinero*, or cook. Depending on the size of the lab, he has anything from two to ten men working for him.

The first stage is to load the leaves into the pit and sprinkle them with lime and water. They are left to stand for several hours to draw the alkaloids out of the leaf. Then kerosene, smuggled from town in big plastic barrels, is added to break the leaves down, and the mixture left for a day or so.

The aim next is to extract the alkaloids from the murky brown mixture and transfer them into the water. This is done by *pisacocas*, or stompers, who walk up and down the pit like hamsters in pairs and 'stomp' the leaves with their bare feet. Usually they are young men who drift to the Chapare from the Altiplano or the city in search of casual work.

The process is usually carried out at night as lab owners know the Leopards rarely carry out patrols after 6.00 p.m. The youths prepare for the gruelling night's work ahead by tanking up with *chicha* (corn beer), or a lethal cocktail of *chicha* and cocaine paste. Miguel, a former stomper, who now sells paste in Cochabamba, describes a night's work:

> You need something inside you to help you *bailar* (dance). We call it dancing because the whole thing turns into a kind of ritual: we stomp the leaves to the rhythm of music which we play on a cassette-recorder. Sometimes it's local Bolivian music. I and my friends prefer American rock.
>
> We keep ourselves going by chewing coca leaves all night. It stops you feeling hungry or thirsty while you are working and keeps you awake. Some guys smoke cocaine paste while they work. Their bosses give it to them as part of their payment: it keeps them in business if they can get the boys addicted. The boys fall into a sort of trance.
>
> We always have two look-outs, young boys with walkie-talkies, who keep an eye out for the police. One stands just beside the *pozo*, the other by the nearest road. If the police arrive the guy by the road radioes the one with us and we leg it into the hills with the *pichicata*. If someone is still at the *pozo* when the police arrive, he says it's an abandoned pit, which I suppose it is.
>
> Usually we work 12-hour stints, but sometimes the boss tells us to carry on until the process is finished. By day we'd crash out in the jungle, if possible on a bamboo bed to avoid the snakes.

Once thoroughly mashed, the mixture is drained. The dead leaves are discarded into a fetid pile beside the pit and the cocaine-rich water, known as *agua rica* (rich water), is siphoned off into large white plastic containers. Sulphuric acid and a touch more lime are then added, making the mixture precipitate and turn milky white.

Finally comes the drying. The mixture is filtered through a big sheet and the precipitate wrapped in toilet paper to extract the moisture; it is left to dry in the sun until it has turned into a greyish clay. This is cocaine paste (about 40 per cent pure cocaine) and in August 1991 it was worth about $250 a kilo, half its 1983 price. According to US estimates, Bolivia produced 575 tonnes of paste in 1990. Other estimates, though, put the figure far higher at around 800 tonnes.

The leftover chemicals, meanwhile, are tipped onto the ground around the pit or into nearby rivers, causing pollution on a devastating scale. Satellite photographs of the region show rivers covered with a purplish oily skin. In villages around Sinahota pollution has become so bad it has made the newly installed water supply unsafe to drink. A report in 1990 by the League for the Defence of the Environment,[4] Bolivia's most respected environmental group, estimated that up to 38,000 tonnes of toxic waste are dumped each year into streams and rivers, which flow into the Amazon network in Brazil. Much of the basin could soon be an ecological disaster zone, it warned.

The most harmful substance is kerosene (paraffin). An estimated three million gallons are dumped each year into the rivers of the Chapare and the Beni. Kerosene, which does not break down chemically, could 'induce massive asphyxiation of aquatic life', said the report. In addition the report estimated that 309 tonnes of sulphuric acid and 7,000 tonnes of calcium sulphate are dumped every year.

Unlike the growing stage, paste processing is very labour intensive. The main labourers are the stompers, who are paid the equivalent in Bolivian currency of between $7 and $15 a night. Sometimes they are paid in cocaine paste. Their pay is a fortune compared with what they would earn in legal jobs, but is around half of what it was in the boom years of the early 1980s. Then, with inflation approaching 24,000 per cent, stompers insisted on being paid in dollars. 'If you got paid in Bolivian money it wasn't worth the trouble,' recalls Miguel. 'You might as well have burned it as waste paper.' But the job has dire costs in terms of health. The chemicals in which the stompers soak their feet leave them cracked and ulcerated. In the early 1980s, Chapare hospitals were packed with stompers whose feet had become so rotten they had to be amputated. Many turned to drugs or prostitution to escape their desperate condition. The stompers also bear the brunt of law enforcement efforts. Often the police will be paid off by big-time traffickers but take home a stomper or two (who cannot afford to make payoffs) to show they have done their job. While the kingpins roam free, stompers cram the prisons in Cochabamba and La Paz.

Apart from the stompers, chemists and look-outs, people are needed to carry out numerous other specific tasks: some collect and transport paste; others liaise with traffickers to have it flown to the Beni; others, known as *chakas* (often women), contract and pay the stompers and provide them with food; another group buys and transports the materials to build the pits, from plastic sheeting to plastic buckets and toilet rolls; others construct them; *zepes* carry precursor chemicals to the pits along secret jungle trails after buying them from middlemen in towns like Sinahota; and so on. For security, people assigned one task know nothing about the rest of the organisation, least of all the name of the top boss.

Hundreds more people in legal or quasi-legal businesses benefit indirectly from the cocaine trade, like hoteliers, restaurant owners and tradesmen selling consumer goods from Sony cassette recorders to bottled beer to gold jewellery. Experts estimate that between 2 and 6 per cent of Bolivia's population profit in some way from the cocaine industry.

MOST of the paste ends up at Isinuta, a sprawling ramshackle jungle town in the heart of the Red Zone from where it is flown to the Beni for further processing. It is a shady unsavoury place. There are so many armed traffickers that, until recently, it was a no-go area for the authorities. Strangers (especially *gringos*) are welcomed with a bullet in the head: that way they ask no questions.

You reach Isinuta by driving a couple of hours up a dirt track which branches off the main Cochabamba to Santa Cruz road just before it reaches Sinahota. Beside the turning, a rusty notice warns drivers that the 'passage of cocaine products or precursor chemicals is strictly forbidden', but is as effective as a 'No litter' sign in London or New York. Two narcotics policemen check passing vehicles, most of them trucks carrying beer or *campesinos*. Beside them strings of young men in denims hang about for no apparent reason. They are the *wokitokeros*, the Spanish rendering of walkie-talkie operators. When a truck load of Leopards or DEA agents turns off to Isinuta, a coded message is sent to another operator 500 metres up the road. 'A canoe is passing', they whisper, canoe being the code for police truck. Or, 'the bloody one is coming', a reference to the truck's red colour. Sometimes the message is an apparently innocuous 'Juan, how are you?' but the next guy along knows it means trouble. Within minutes traffickers in Isinuta have been warned and have fled to their jungle hide-outs with their dope. Often the look-outs are young boys; they can be paid less, and being under age cannot be arrested.

Quiet by day, at night Isinuta buzzes with activity. The traffickers tell the town they are ready for business by firing a few gunshots. At the signal, villagers take their plastic bags of paste to the appointed collection point. This is usually an abandoned house on the outskirts, or a private house that the druglords hire for the night. A girl whose boyfriend, Jaime, buys and sells paste in Isinuta described his work:

> Jaime begins selling at around 9.00 p.m. and carries on until around midnight, depending on how much business there is. When the price of coca leaf is low, business falls too. Jaime picked up the tricks of the trade working for somebody else, but now he works on his own. It's much safer. If you work with other people you never know when they might turn you in. He enjoys the work, it's exciting. It pays well too; that's why he takes the risk. Luckily he hasn't been caught yet. Just in case, he carries arms. The boss gives him automatic weapons in exchange for cocaine paste.

The busiest days of the month are days of *cobertura* or cover, specific days when the police have been paid off to allow the traffickers to land their small planes without interference. 'The word gets around as to when and where the traffickers are going to pick up the paste,' says one Isinuta inhabitant who calls himself Fernando. 'One month it will be Isinuta, the next it may be another town like Eteramazama. On those days everyone is frantically busy. They abandon their crops and rush with their paste to the collection point.'

With a combination of coercion and riches, the *narcos* have little problem winning the allegiance of Isinuta's inhabitants. 'People like the *narcos* because they provide them with a living,' says Jaime's girlfriend.

The same does not go for the Leopards, who are universally hated. Poor and uneducated, they see anti-drug patrols and raids as opportunities to make a quick killing. In Eteramazama, 40 minutes' drive from Isinuta, the owner of the village restaurant has to close at dusk because the Leopards seized the diesel he brought by road to work his generator. One Christmas Day the Leopards filched $10,000 from the offices of the local cooperative, which had been collected to finish the building of a school. 'They had an excellent Christmas party,' says the leader of the local peasant union.

In the nearby town of Chimoré things are even worse, as one woman recounts:

One day in March 1990 the DEA and UMOPAR did a joint raid on all the houses in Chimoré. They knocked on our door at 5.00 a.m. When we didn't open, they just kicked it down and forced their way in. My daughter was on her own downstairs doing her homework. I was still in bed upstairs. 'Why did you come to the Chapare?' they asked her. They opened all the drawers and helped themselves to anything they wanted, even my daughter's bras and knickers.

If a woman is on her own, they rape her. If she makes a fuss, they drag her off to the police station. They make her hand over her jewellery, even her wedding ring.

Just because we live in Chimoré they treat us like *narcos*. But we didn't choose to be here. It's an impossible situation. If we say we've got nothing to say they say we must be involved in drugs. When we go past a checkpoint carrying toilet paper they take it, even if it's obviously just for the house. The police ought to protect us. Instead, we need to be protected from them.

Three years ago the Leos killed a man from here. To keep his wife quiet they bought her the newspaper kiosk on the corner. It's still there, only it's closed because she can't afford to stock it.

When inhabitants of Chimoré go to Cochabamba it is just as bad. 'Simply being from the Chapare makes them suspicious,' says a spokesman for the Cochabamba-based Permanent Assembly for Human Rights.

They are taken to the narcotics police headquarters and have all their possessions taken from them, including their car and money. They are beaten and told to hand over their cocaine paste, even if they don't have any. The police make it clear that the only way they will get out is by paying, so their families are forced to go away and get the money together. Two or three people are picked up like this every week.

In 1991 tensions in the Chapare increased after the government, under pressure from the US, agreed to involve the Bolivian army in the fight against drugs and began forcibly to eradicate coca plantations which had been newly planted. *Chapareños* warned that if pushed against the wall Bolivia's *campesinos* could become a fertile breeding ground for insurgent groups like Peru's Shining Path. They responded to the government's decision to involve the army by setting up self-defence committees, which they claim are armed.

In August the atmosphere deteriorated further when police shot and killed a coca farmer after a group of growers attacked officials who were trying to destroy illegal coca plantations as part of an intensified eradication campaign: 300 hectares were destroyed in the Chapare in July and August 1991 alone. Several Ministry of Agriculture officials were injured.

THE COCA boom began in the 1970s as a result of soaring demand from consumers, mainly in the US, who could not stuff the white powder up their noses fast enough. But the leaf has been cultivated in South America for at least 2,000 years, chewed by indigenous Indians to help them endure the punishing conditions in which they live. A mild stimulant, coca fulfils much the same function as cigarettes and alcohol in the West.

Under the Inca empire coca was probably a privilege reserved for the royal family and priests (although historians disagree about this) and specific communities were charged with its cultivation. After the Spanish conquest, however, anybody could buy the leaves and the habit of chewing rapidly caught on. Coca was used extensively in heathen rites and almost worshipped for its seemingly magical powers as a stimulant. Coca chewers found they could go for days without eating, drinking or sleeping.

The Spaniards realised huge profits were to be made from this wonder plant. 'There has never been in the whole world a plant or root or any growing thing that bears and yields every year as this does... or that is so highly valued,' wrote one chronicler, Pedro Cieza de León, early in the 16th century. The natives were dragged from their highland hovels to work in steamy lowland plantations. Many could not take the climate and died. Others caught diseases which their weak bodies were defenceless to fight. Contemporary historians estimate that between a third and a half of the annual quota of coca-workers died after their five-month service. As the chronicler Hernando de Santillán put it, 'down there [in the coca plantations] there is one disease worse than all the rest: the unrestrained greed of the Spaniards.'[5]

The popularity of the coca leaf, however, worried the Spanish ecclesiastics who feared it was an obstacle to the spread of Christianity. 'Coca is a plant that the devil invented for the total destruction of the natives,' wrote one, called Diego de Robles. But the ecclesiastics' views clashed with those of Spanish merchants who discovered that if you gave Indian workers leaves to chew you didn't need to feed them and they put in double the hours. *Mitayos*, Indian workers press-ganged into working in Bolivia's silver mines, were paid in coca. Realising coca's advantages, Viceroy Toledo in 1573 gave up trying to beat the problem and taxed it instead.

The habit of chewing continues today. In the silver mines of Potosí, high in the Altiplano, miners see their little plastic bags of coca leaves as essential as their pick-axes and oil lamps. Seated in silent rows outside the mine entrances on Potosí's *Cerro Rico* (Rich Hill), they start chewing at dawn to calm their nerves. Every day someone is swallowed up into the mountain's pitch-black entrails after being crushed by an avalanche of falling rock. Each miner just hopes it will not be him. One miner, called Jorge, describes the role of coca in his life:

> My wife gets up at four o'clock and cooks breakfast (usually rice and milk and perhaps some coffee) which we eat at around six. I leave for work at seven and stop at the bottom of the Cerro to buy my coca leaves. They come from the Yungas, they are sweeter than the Chapare leaves. I buy about two ounces a day, which costs me around one *boliviano* [30 US cents], that's around a tenth of what I earn in a day. When I reach the mine entrance we chew for half an hour to give us strength for the day before starting at nine.
>
> Down the mine we chew leaves all day to keep us going. Because of all the dust and gas we can't eat so the leaves stop us getting hungry. Coca helps you bear the life down there. I find myself a face where I can find some veins of silver. Apart from the sound of distant tapping, it's as silent and dark as the grave. The further down you go the hotter it gets. When you work on the lower levels, it can reach 45 degrees, so you have to strip to your underpants.

Coca is also still an integral part of the lives of thousands of Quechua and Aymara Indians who scrape a living herding sheep and llamas on the high Altiplano. It serves as a powerful symbol of their cultural identity. In rural areas of Bolivia virtually every labourer carries a little pouch (or *k'intus*) of leaves in his pocket. In rural communities coca chewing, known as *acullicu*, is seen as an essential social skill in much the same way as drinking is seen in the West. Adults chew it after meals and pause for 'coca breaks', just as Westerners stop for smoking breaks. Leaves are still used in rituals, such as blessing a new house, and for medicinal purposes to cure anything from a cold to tuberculosis to a broken leg.

Coca is consumed by chewing the leaves and holding them in the cheek in a ball. To the leaves is added a little grey stone, like pumice, made of vegetable ash which helps release the alkaloids, of which cocaine is one. The cocaine alkaloid is absorbed into the bloodstream through the mouth's mucous membrane, slightly numbing the cheeks and acting as a mild stimulant on the body. The dose of cocaine in the leaves, however, is minuscule and there is no evidence that coca leaf is addictive. The difference between chewing coca and snorting cocaine is as great as the difference between riding a donkey and flying Concorde.

In Bolivia's cities, where the middle classes view chewing as a dirty rural habit, coca still serves an important use as tea or *maté*. Every tourist who has suffered the unpleasant effects of altitude sickness in La Paz or Potosí, both over 12,000 feet above sea level, is familiar with the alleviating effects of the spinach-tasting yellow *maté de coca*. The capital's smartest hotels serve it. Officials at the US embassy in downtown La Paz offer visitors coca tea as they explain the vital need for eradication. When the Pope visited La Paz in 1986 the local press published daily accounts of how many cups of coca tea he drank.

Ironically, the cocaine industry is bad news for Bolivia's estimated 1.5 million chewers. Coca growers prefer to sell to traffickers than to legal government wholesalers, who pay far less. As a result, little is left for the local market. What is tends to be expensive and of shoddy quality, especially after police have disrupted traffickers' operations. Chewers complain they can only afford to buy dusty 'left-overs' which no-one else wants. Some have turned to alcohol, like *chicha* or beer, instead.

Coca's role as a stimulant and as a symbol of cultural identity is used by coca farmers to defend the cultivation of coca leaf against elimination by 'imperialist' forces. The sacred leaf is as much part of Bolivian culture as hamburgers are of US culture, they argue, and no outsiders have a right to destroy it. Their views are voiced by powerful coca growers' unions which, unlike California's shadowy marijuana growers who have no public profile, are a legal 'up front' force with considerable political clout. The largest Chapare union is led by Evo Morales, an elusive unsmiling man whose defence of the coca leaf is as passionate as his hatred of journalists and *gringos*, particularly those who work at The Embassy (US of course). Like the militant miners' unions, the coca unions use highly effective but peaceful mass mobilisation tactics like sit-ins, hunger strikes and road blocks to make themselves heard.

Even in the Chapare, where coca is patently not grown for traditional uses, coca farmers react furiously when US officials or journalists suggest they are criminals, drug addicts or traffickers. An article in *Newsweek* in 1986,[6] for example, captioned a photograph of a woman selling coca leaves in a market with the words 'Harvest of Shame'. Growers argue that they simply grow the leaf to make a living and sell to whoever pays the highest price (as any sensible farmer would). How it is then used is none of their business. As one US official put it, 'These people are not addicted to coca, they are addicted to eating.'

The credibility of the farmers' arguments, however, is often undermined by the fact that many *cocaleros* (and allegedly their leaders too) are also involved in the illegal cocaine industry. The reasons why peasants have become involved (usually a combination of coercion and economic necessity) and their resentment at being used as scapegoats for the activities of the drug barons are understandable. But the refusal of union leaders to admit that some of their members work in the cocaine industry does not further their cause. This reluctance to admit the truth was noticeable at a meeting of Andean coca growers in La Paz in March 1991. One group at the meeting was asked to discuss the relation between coca and cocaine, but its members refused to admit they knew anything at all about the cocaine industry and instead spent two days discussing coca. Every time the word 'cocaine' was mentioned, two Indian women in the back row yelled, 'We don't know anything about that. We just grow coca.'

WHATEVER the traditional virtues of the coca leaf, US politicians in the mid-1980s decided that all Bolivia's coca, except for the small amount needed for its chewers, must go. The eradication of South America's coca fields became the obsession of the US's anti-drug warriors. Under US pressure, Bolivian governments established and then failed to implement a series of eradication agreements drawn up with the US embassy. Bolivian politicians knew the accords would never work, and perhaps some did not want them to, but they knew that if they wanted US aid they had to sign on the dotted line.

The most radical piece of legislation was the Coca Law, approved after months of haggling in July 1988. For the first time in Bolivia's history, the cultivation of coca was defined as illegal except for 12,000 hectares in the Yungas for domestic consumption. The rest of Bolivia's coca was defined as 'excess' and was to be eradicated at a rate of between 5,000 and 8,000 hectares a year. Overnight, the majority of Bolivia's coca farmers had turned into social delinquents.

The Coca Law was a victory for the US, which had drafted most of the text. But Washington did not get its way totally; under pressure from the coca unions, the Bolivian government banned the use of herbicides and defoliants to wipe out coca. They also lost on the issue of compensation: since coca was now illegal, US officials did not think growers should be compensated. But at the unions' insistence the government agreed that all eradication in transitional areas like the Chapare should be voluntary and that farmers would be paid $2,000 a hectare. When a farmer wanted to eradicate, he would notify DIRECO, the Bolivian eradication agency, which would monitor the process and arrange compensation.

The following year, 1989, Bolivia, as in all previous years, failed to meet the eradication targets set for it by the US government. A meagre 2,500 hectares of coca were destroyed, half the US target. It was only just more than the area of new coca that was planted.

In 1990 the situation changed dramatically. This was not because coca growers had suddenly decided they agreed with eradication, but because the price of the coca leaf dropped through the floor. Having sold at around $85 in August 1989, by April 1990 a *carga* could not fetch more than $10, less than it cost to produce. Coca farmers rushed to DIRECO's offices in Villa Tunari. 'We've got a stampede going and we've got to take advantage, or excuses aren't going to hold,' the DEA's country attaché, Don Ferrarone, told reporters in May 1990. Officials at an agricultural extension centre complained they could not cope. 'Coca farmers can't get out of coca fast enough. So many people are volunteering to switch to other crops that we can't deal with them,' said one. In April alone, farmers had wiped out 1,000 hectares of coca, nearly half the amount eradicated in the whole of the previous year. By the end of the year they had destroyed over 8,000, well over the annual target.

Narcotics experts in La Paz traded theories as to why the price had dropped. US diplomats said it was the result of a successful clamp-down against drug traffickers in Colombia. With no-one to buy coca leaves, the price had slumped. Some Bolivian officials had another view. The price of the leaf had dropped because too many people were still growing coca. The price slump, they said, was the result of overproduction.

JULIANO Méndez is one of the farmers who has decided to get out of coca. Standing outside his house in a hamlet called Senda Tres (Road Three) with his wife and two tiny daughters, he watches a red DIRECO land cruiser stop on the dirt track in front. At 7.00 a.m. on 21 July 1990 D-Day has finally arrived.

Watched suspiciously by his wife, Juliano shakes hands with the DIRECO team boss, a man named Víctor Candia, and leads the group through a field of coca bushes and banana trees and over a rushing river which they cross with stepping stones. A few hundred yards along a tiny path, they reach a field of coca. Four labourers are hacking the bushes with axes and machetes. To minimise his losses, Juliano harvested them a few days earlier.

Juliano decided to destroy his coca crop when the price dropped to $10. 'It wasn't worth bothering to take the leaves to the market. The price is now $27 but I've decided to get out.' But eradicating the fields is not cheap. He has to pay his workers five *bolivianos* ($1.70) a day, and meals on top. It will take them around 18 days to eradicate the whole field.

The future is uncertain. Juliano's $2,000 compensation will last two or three months. He will be able to pay off some debts and buy food and shoes for the family. 'Maybe we will have to go and live in Cochabamba,' he says. 'It is cheaper there.' Alternatively, although he won't say it, he may move deeper into the jungle and plant new illegal coca.

He looks sadly at his dead coca bushes as if they were the corpses of his children. 'It seems such a shame. Money is all very well, but it doesn't last. Coca, on the other hand, is a long-term investment.' He is doubtful whether he will get his compensation straight away; friends of his who had eradicated their coca fields had had to wait three or four months for payment. Even then the officials usually find reasons to reduce the amount, arguing, for example, that some of the coca was newly planted.

But Juliano's biggest worry is what will replace his coca. 'I planted mandarin trees six years ago, so hopefully I will be able to live off those. But the prices I get for them are a joke: three *bolivianos* [$1] for 100. That's once they've reached Cochabamba. About a quarter of them rot on the way.'

Although Juliano has decided it is time to get out of coca, his wife, Rosa, is dead against it. Watching distraught as the workmen destroy her family's livelihood, she turns angrily to Víctor. 'How are we going to live now? Now we're stuck here without coca, are we going to live off insects? It costs ten *bolivianos* [$3] just to pay the bus fare to Villa Tunari. I spend 100 [$35] a month on food.'

Víctor finishes writing down the measurements of Juliano's plot in his notebook and signals to his men to return to the truck. 'I'll come back in a month to check the coca has all been destroyed. Leave one coca bush in the middle of the field so that we can prove it was coca.'

SIX months later the stampede to destroy coca had fizzled out. The reason: the coca price had crept up again. By October 1990, it had returned to $70 a *carga* and stayed there for the first half of 1991. Coca farmers who had joined the unemployed in Cochabamba returned to their fields in the Chapare. Those who had destroyed theirs worked for friends, stomped coca or planted fresh coca plantations further afield. The price fall, hailed by US officials as a sign that their policies were working, appeared to have been just another turn in the ebb and flow of supply and demand. In fact the depression had probably had the opposite effect from that intended: unable to survive by growing coca leaf, many had turned to making paste instead.

The biggest problem was that the price fall did not last long enough to give alternative crops a chance. According to the DEA, for the coca price to affect people's willingness to change, it must remain low for between 12 and 14 months, an impossibility. In Washington Senator Joe Biden had urged the US administration to respond to the price fall by giving $125 million in emergency aid to the farmers. But the bureaucrats, who had neatly apportioned US aid on a five-year basis, said their plans could not be changed. No extra aid was sent. When the price went up again, Biden was furious. 'The administration has been slow in responding to the changing circumstances in the international drug trade,' he said. 'As a result, the US and the Andean countries may have missed a[n]... opportunity to convince a substantial number of coca farmers in South America to grow other crops.'[7]

While the policy makers bickered, coca farmers in the Chapare complained that there were no alternatives to switch to. 'The government says it believes in eradication together with development. So far we've seen plenty of eradication but no development,' says Evo Morales. 'In 1990 the government spent about $12 million on destroying coca fields but USAID spent only $2.5 million on projects to develop alternative crops. Now they've eradicated their coca fields, farmers have nothing to grow. Many wish they'd hung onto their coca.'

Bodies like USAID, which are trying to develop new crops, have been long on promises but short on solutions, he says. The crops are being developed at two agricultural research stations run jointly by USAID and the Bolivian Institute for Agricultural Technology (IBTA). There are traditional crops, like maize and rice, plus almost every non-traditional crop you can think of, from passion fruit to ginger to pineapples. There are even macadamia nuts and palms flown over specially from Costa Rica. In theory farmers should plant a selection of different crops so that harvests can be spread over the year. With crops like macadamia, which take up to eight years to produce, maize, rice or bananas can be planted in the meantime. To get started, farmers are offered a two-year credit through the Bank of Cochabamba.

Unfortunately, the reality has not been that simple. Plants like macadamia which had been flown in from abroad were so expensive that no-one could afford them. The stations' carefully tended rows of exotic plants bloomed undisturbed, prompting one critic to dub them 'the best botanical gardens in the Chapare'. At the La Jota station, near Chimoré, officials had to slash the price to get local farmers interested. 'We started selling macadamia at $26 a plant but no-one bought them,' says station director Francisco Zannier. 'So now we're selling them at $13.'

The earnings farmers were promised they would make with their new crops also turned out to be illusory. When farmers bought passion fruit plants, for example, they were promised an income of $1,600 per hectare, according to Carlos Balderrama, adviser to Evo Morales. He says they actually earn a tenth of that. The drop in earnings was not of course the fault of the agricultural station but the result of fluctuations in world commodity prices. Crops that are valuable one year may be worthless the next, as René Navajas, the director of a former project run by the United Nations Fund for Drug Abuse Control (UNFDAC) in the Yungas, found to his cost. 'When we started the project we persuaded the farmers to grow coffee because the price was excellent,' he said in 1990. 'Now it has dropped to a third of what it was and the farmers are accusing us of deceiving them.'

And although most farmers welcomed the idea of credits, in the end only 5 per cent of those who had wiped out their coca got them. The interest, 13 per cent, was so high that many did not even apply because they knew no crop would ever give them that kind of return. Many who did apply found they were ineligible because to qualify they had to possess some guarantees, such as a house in town or some livestock (land, being free, does not count). In effect only the wealthier farmers were eligible. Also, the maximum duration of credits of under $5,000 was two years. It was a mystery how farmers who had chosen to plant macadamia, which takes eight years to produce, were to pay the money back.

Farmers are hampered too by transport, or lack of it. Both the Chapare and the Yungas are extremely difficult to reach by road. Unlike coca, which is collected at the farm gate, other products must be driven for several hours at considerable expense along tortuous roads to reach the nearest market. The transport problem has prompted some development agencies like UNFDAC to focus increasingly on agro-industries, like small factories to produce tea, glucose and yuca-based animal feed, and on basic infrastructure projects such as roads, bridges and electricity. The British government has put £2.2 million into a UNFDAC project to provide hundreds of households with drinking water. Without these, attempts to diversify into other crops or agro-industries have little chance of success.

UNFDAC has constructed nearly 300 kilometres of roads in the Chapare. But that has a serious snag: the roads are used by drug traffickers as landing strips. In fact, that was the reason USAID scrapped its road-building projects in the mid-1980s and let the DEA blow up the roads.

A recent incident illustrates the problems. The day in March 1991 that UNFDAC opened a 15-kilometre section of road between Santa Rosa and Puerto Trinitario, to the east of Isinuta, the traffickers threw a *fiesta*. At six o'clock the next morning the first trafficking plane landed, picked up its white powder cargo and took off again five minutes later. At eight o'clock another tried to land but crashed into a mandarin tree. The traffickers grabbed the plane engine and radios and fled, leaving the charred wreck strewn across the road. The next day peasant leaders banged wooden posts into the middle of the road to make it unusable as an airstrip, but were threatened by traffickers who promised to retaliate. 'What are we to do?' asks Jaime Idrovo, head of UNFDAC's Chapare projects. 'Do we stop building roads simply because the traffickers might use them? They only need 300 metres of road to land their planes. Do we prevent development reaching these people in case it falls into the wrong hands? I believe not. Such a strategy is like saying you won't buy your child some decent-sized shoes because you don't want him to grow up.'

Even if farmers do get their produce to market, there is no guarantee that anyone will buy it, either at home or abroad. One woman, for example, who produced her own passion fruit juice found locals unwilling to switch from Coca Cola and Sprite which were more familiar to them. Coffee producers have found the Bolivian public reluctant to substitute home-grown fresh coffee for imported instant. In another example, two private producers and USAID/IBTA produced 60 tonnes of ginger only to find that no-one would buy it.[8]

Bolivian produce is often of too poor a quality to compete on the international market, in some cases because farmers see pesticides and fertilisers as expensive extras rather than essentials. Another drawback is that producers lack the technology to package their goods. Producers of oranges, for example, which grow well in the Chapare, could make a good business if they could turn them into canned orange juice or concentrate, but no canning factory has yet been built.

Abroad, Bolivian exports face high import duties. In the view of many development experts, removal of these tariffs is one of the most useful contributions industrialised countries could make to fighting the production of cocaine in South America. The European Community has already taken some important steps in this direction by abolishing tariffs on most farm exports from Bolivia, Peru, Ecuador and Colombia for four years until 1994 and scrapping duties on industrial goods. In 1990 the US Congress proposed an Andean Trade Preferences Act, but by mid-1991 this had still not yet been approved.

One of the biggest obstacles facing Bolivian farmers wishing to switch from coca to other crops is the US farm lobby. In particular, attempts by Bolivia to export soya have met strong opposition from US soya farmers who say US economic aid should not be used to promote crops which compete with US ones. In summer 1990 the dispute flared up into a full-blown row between the US State Department, whose anti-drugs policy included support for crop substitution, and the US Agriculture Department, which supported the farmers. The matter was only solved after Robert Gelbard, the US ambassador to Bolivia, intervened personally in support of the State Department and pointed out that the 52,000 tonnes of soybean which Bolivia planned to export in 1990 was derisory compared with the 17 million tonnes produced by the US.

Inside Bolivia, foreign-financed development programmes are viewed with deep suspicion by coca farmers and their unions, who, historically wary of outsiders, also see them as the soft end of repressive anti-drugs policies. US-funded projects, for example, make a direct link between development and eradication. Communities and individuals must destroy 30 per cent of their coca fields to be eligible for a development project, 60 per cent for two and so on. 'Linking development assistance to eradication was the only way we could get any money from Washington,' explains one USAID official in La Paz. 'We had to convince sceptical congressmen back home who didn't even know where Bolivia was. They had to see that their money was having a direct effect on the amount of coca grown.' Coca leaders, on the other hand, argue that development is a human right and should not be conditional on anything. In the case of USAID projects, they also complain that too much emphasis is put on 'immediate-impact' projects like schools and clinics at the expense of funding for alternative crops. 'Schools and clinics are very nice, but we can't eat them,' comments one coca farmer. 'They don't solve the problem of how we are going to survive when we've destroyed our coca.'

The problem with making development projects conditional on eradication is that it makes it hard to develop a long-term development plan for the region. Instead, it tends to lead to *ad hoc* dubious, unconnected projects in inappropriate places. A *campesino* market, for example, was built in Chimoré at a cost of $9,000 because inhabitants had agreed to destroy 100 per cent of their coca crop. Sadly, the town already had a permanent market with 150 stalls of which only 25 were used.[9] Another project provided bricks for the construction of part of a prison, although what connection a prison had with development was a mystery. Almost no development projects, on the other hand, have been set up in the best agricultural lands to the east since these coincide with the Red Zone, the heart of the Chapare's cocaine industry. In the case of US-funded development projects, planning is made yet more difficult by the fact that half of US economic assistance to Bolivia is held up for at least six months pending the president giving his stamp of approval by 'certifying' Bolivia, and tends to have political strings attached.

Aid experts are increasingly concluding that crop substitution in the Chapare is a lost cause. As long as there is demand for cocaine, coca will always pay more than any other crop, sometimes as much as 20 times more. The Chapare's poor soils and high rainfall also make it unsuitable for many alternatives. It is difficult, too, to provide coca farmers with compensation and development projects without having the unwanted effect of increasing their income and economic security (particularly as many take compensation and plant new coca) which gives them little incentive to seek jobs elsewhere, and may even attract farmers from other areas who may later turn to coca.

Many aid experts now believe that rather than 'pushing' farmers out of coca by giving them compensation, they should be 'pulled' to areas outside the Chapare, particularly the highlands. In other words, rather than replacing the individual coca plants, it is better to make the Bolivian economy as a whole less dependent on cocaine. If projects in regions like the highlands are successful, peasants in the Chapare, many of whom originate from there, will hopefully return. Highlanders who might have migrated to the Chapare would stay at home.

This thinking prompted USAID in 1987 to set up its High Valley project in the Cochabamba Department, from where many *Chapareños* come. This included irrigation and drinking water projects, road construction and forestry. A similar project has been set up by the European Community near Potosí. 'Our earlier approach was too narrow,' says Darell McIntyre, a USAID official in La Paz. 'We attempted substitution when the price of coca was sky high. Nothing could compete with that so the projects flopped. Now we see our role as providing alternatives to coca anywhere in the country. This may mean working as a tailor in Potosí or growing potatoes in the Cochabamba Valley.' The biggest problem, he says, is convincing people back home that projects like this constitute coca substitution. 'They couldn't understand why we were funding projects in areas where there was no coca. Now they are slowly coming round to the idea.' The drawback with such projects is that they do little to dissuade coca farmers from growing coca and offer nothing for *Chapareños* who want to change crops but do not wish to leave their homes. For the projects to be effective, peasants would have to be moved forcibly, which is clearly an impossibility.

Whatever the solution, it will have to be long term. The problem is that Washington and European countries, which provide the funds, want quick results or will lose interest. As one US official confided, 'The process will take a generation. But we don't tell that to people in Washington who want a quick fix. We tell them it will be done by next year.' Many farmers in the Chapare, tired of being harassed by police and traffickers alike, would like a quick fix too. They know that demand for coca will not last for ever. But until something else comes along, coca will continue to spread its roots ever deeper into Bolivia's rain forests.

3

Kings of Cocaine:
The Traffickers

Santa Cruz

IN the tropical heat of midday, Santa Cruz's Plaza de 24 Septiembre slumps into a lethargic doze. Armies of ragamuffin shoeshine boys clutching their wooden boxes of assorted brushes and polishes weave in and out of the palm trees and the colonial-style arcades in search of a willing pair of feet. On the benches round the central fountain, plain clothes police in dark glasses and immaculately ironed shirts idly watch passers-by. Beside them, ancient photographers with even more ancient box cameras on tripods plunge under large black blankets to photograph rows of schoolgirls in white school uniforms like dentists' coats. In the well-heeled residential districts on the outskirts of the city, the quiver of a guard's pistol and the bleep of a short-wave radio are the only signs of life.

But the sleepy tranquillity of this jungle city, Bolivia's second largest, is deceptive. Behind the closed doors and the dark glasses is being conducted the country's most profitable business: cocaine.

Located strategically between the coca fields of the Chapare and the cocaine-processing laboratories of the Beni, and equipped with a glossy international airport, Santa Cruz is the headquarters of Bolivia's drugs industry.

It is also the home of the country's largest traffickers. Almost all the big names have their town houses here or did so once, including Techo de Paja (Thatch Roof) and his uncle, Roberto Suárez, known as the 'King of Cocaine'. Most live in exclusive residential areas like Equipetrol, five kilometres north of the centre, a sort of Bolivian Beverly Hills which took its name from a US oil equipment company which once did business here. Surrounded by spike-studded brick walls and gorgeous pink bougainvillea, the luxury terracotta-roofed mansions are so vast each one could be a little college. Their unique style of discreet opulence has given rise to a new mode of architecture which the locals call *narco-arquitectura*. The drug barons rub elbows with politicians: General Hugo Banzer, a former right-wing military dictator who heads one of the parties in the governing coalition, has his country residence in Equipetrol. Outside, guards keep watch from little white pillboxes. On the pavement imported BMWs and Mercedes shimmer in the sun. There is even a Rolls Royce, almost certainly the only one in Bolivia. Its ignition keys, so local legend has it, are made of pure gold.

Inside, flanked by bodyguards, the traffickers conduct business, or take it easy by the pool. If they are big fry they do not go into the street, especially if they know they are being looked for. But under the cover of night, they go to restaurants or discotheques with their bodyguards.

One of their favourite eating places is La Herradura, an exclusive steak house owned by an Iranian. For a change, they go to El Buen Gusto (Good Taste). Ironically, both are also favourite hangouts for US DEA agents. One agent enjoys telling the story of how, one Sunday evening, he went into La Herradura to find himself face to face with Bolivia's most wanted trafficker at the time, Techo de Paja, and three bodyguards. Being Sunday though, neither could do anything about the other, and in any case DEA agents are not authorised to shoot or make arrests. 'He was not on duty that day, and neither was I,' says the agent, 'so we nodded politely.'

Although the *narcotraficantes* take their bodyguards everywhere, security is not an overwhelming problem: regular 'don't touch me' payments to local police, and friendship ties, ensure virtual immunity. Locals see the druglords walk in and out of the police station without turning a hair. In 1990 the going rate was $52,000 a month, not a bad incentive for a policeman who would otherwise earn between $60 and $100. Not surprisingly, police jobs in Santa Cruz are the most sought after in Bolivia. According to a DEA source, police colonels pay up to $250,000 for the position of head of the Santa Cruz narcotics police.

Together with oil money (rich oil fields were discovered here in the 1970s) cocaine wealth has turned what used to be a forgotten dirt-street jungle town into Bolivia's richest city. With its high-rise blocks, elegant cocktail bars and international airport, Santa Cruz is a world apart from the barren towns of the impoverished Altiplano. Even the people are different: *cruceños* (as the locals are called) are famous for their happy-go-lucky attitude to life, their riotous festivals and incongruous blue eyes. Their music too, in contrast to the mournful tones of the Andes, is imbued with the throbbing rhythms of Africa and Brazil. This is the heart of Bolivia's Wild West.

A trained eye can spot the imprint of the coke trade everywhere. You will see more Mercedes and Mitsubishi jeeps here than in stockbroker Surrey. In fact, Bolivia has the highest number of luxury cars per capita in Latin America, quite extraordinary when you consider that the country is also South America's poorest. You will find clothes that you would not find in Paris (at half the price) and rings with precious stones as big as golf balls.

Santa Cruz is where cocaine dollars are fronted. Traffickers used to stash them in tax havens like Panama or the Cayman Islands or invest them in Miami properties, but recent banking investigations have made them nervous. Many now prefer to keep at least part of their wealth in Bolivia, whose liberal banking laws ensure no questions are asked. They launder it in Santa Cruz by setting up businesses like discotheques, restaurants, estate agents or car or small aeroplane dealerships. They sell the planes, usually Cessna 206s, to fellow traffickers who park them in rows at Santa Cruz's domestic airport. The cars are smuggled from Brazil or Chile, with a few wads of greenbacks ensuring customs officers ask no questions at the border. They sell at a fraction of the price in the country they are made. You can pick up a Suzuki Jeep, for example, for a mere $15,000, and a Mercedes Benz for around $25,000. The businesses often run at a loss. But at least they give vast fortunes a legal look about them and distract the attention of police or DEA agents who might otherwise ask questions.

Until recently, cocaine was so much part of *cruceño* life that the *narcos* scarcely bothered to hide their assets. Every *cruceño* knew who owned what. It was common knowledge, for example, that the Number One supermarket was owned by Techo de Paja and another, Extra, is still owned by Erwin Gasser, another suspected trafficker. Techo de Paja's *hacienda*, El Horizonte, opposite Santa Cruz airport, was well known by locals until it was seized, although few had been inside. It had thoroughbred horses imported from Saudi Arabia and Hereford cows from Britain. They knew his town house, too, which had a swimming pool and chandeliers from Miami. And it was an open secret that hot money lay behind a $3 million discotheque called Reginne's, a favourite nightspot for US tourists. It was owned by an up-and-coming trafficker called Carmelo 'Meco' Domínguez. Technically, Reginne's was registered in the name of Domínguez's doctor and the discotheque's amiable manageress would inform guests with a smile that it was owned by a 'limited company'. Unfortunately for Domínguez, documents and computer records which police found when they raided it in 1990 left them in no doubt that he was the real owner.

Even one of the city's basketball teams runs on narcodollars, according to one of its coaches. Owned by a wealthy trafficker, it hires a couple of Americans as players or coaches. `We get paid $2,500 a month. It's easy money, although the standards aren't very high so you get a bit rusty,' says its black American coach, a lanky seven foot four. 'The owner of the team invites Americans down and has a look at them. He sends them back if he doesn't like them. The team is only allowed two Americans at a time. Being here gives you good contacts if you want to dabble in dope. I don't buy the stuff myself, but my team leader is a dealer.' Local football teams, like Blooming and Destroyers, have also done well out of cocaine: traffickers buy professional players and give them to the teams. In return they are treated with the respect due to a feudal lord.

Apart from being an investment centre, Santa Cruz is where traffickers do business. 'It's their command and control centre where all the arrangements and deals are made,' says a DEA source. Gathered in offices in the buildings of their fabricated businesses, or in the safety of their homes, traffickers meet their buyers and distributors and fix when and where a shipment of finished cocaine will be picked up from a lab. They arrange pilots. Sometimes they don't tell the pilots the exact location until they are airborne in case they decide to earn extra money by informing. The buyers tend to be Argentinians or Brazilians who stay in the city's scores of luxury hotels. From Santa Cruz, too, traffickers arrange for their money to be hidden in foreign bank accounts. They avoid Miami and Panama, preferring Switzerland and Chile.

Cocaine is run much like any other business and until recently no social stigma was attached to those who dealt in it. In fact some come from the city's oldest sugar and tin oligarchy families. There are self-starters too, like 'Meco' Domínguez who began as a used-car dealer. *Cruceños* are long accustomed to asking no questions. Not even the druglords' wives. 'Often traffickers do not tell their wives what business they are in, or how much they earn,' says a DEA source. 'They live as any respectable family, their kids go to school, they go to the club at weekends.'

In 1986 something happened to change those attitudes. It involved the director of Santa Cruz' Botanical and Zoological Garden, a few blocks down from Equipetrol. His name was Noel Kempff. An enthusiastic botanist and zoologist, he made regular trips into the jungles near Santa Cruz to collect specimens. On 5 September 1986, after landing his plane on a rough airstrip in the Huanchaca National Park, northeast of Santa Cruz, he and his three companions came under a hail of machine-gun fire: they had stumbled across one of the country's largest cocaine laboratories, reportedly owned by Techo de Paja, or a *cruceño* family called Chavez. Three men, including Kempff, died immediately. The fourth, a Spaniard, was miraculously spotted by a rescue plane the next day and survived to tell the story. Thousands of *cruceños* who flocked to the funeral wept as they were played some of the recordings that Kempff had made of birds in the jungle to make the ones in the zoo feel more at home. Today, a statue of Kempff outside the zoo is a poignant reminder of the ruthlessness of the traffickers. 'From then on, *cruceños* couldn't kid themselves any more that the *narcos* were decent normal people,' says a resident. 'They could be ruthless killers too. People began to avoid them if they could.'

Clubs like the exclusive Equestrian Club in Santa Cruz did not want to be seen with well-known traffickers on their books and quietly asked them to leave. They were reluctant at first, nervous about how the drug barons might react. But when a Bolivian general, Gary Prado, one of their oldest and most prestigious members, threatened to quit unless the barons were expelled, they got a move on. Even the city's Civic Committee, a sort of town council, has cleared out some traffickers after consulting with the DEA.

SANTA Cruz was founded in 1561 by a weary rabble of Spaniards who had spent months trekking across the desolate plains of the Paraguayan Chaco. The region's combination of grassland savannah and jungle at the foothills of the *sierra* made it an ideal location. The Spaniards cut down the forest and built a mini Spanish city, complete with colonial-style arcades and a fine salmon-pink cathedral overlooking a central plaza. For centuries Santa Cruz was isolated from the rest of Bolivia until, in the 1950s, the government built a road to Cochabamba and a railway to Brazil. These attracted hordes of immigrants, from highlander Indians in black and red handwoven robes escaping the cold of the Andes to tall Mennonites in denim dungarees and wide-brimmed straw hats from Canada and the US who set up as farmers. Settlers even came from Japan to grow cotton, rice and coffee.

It was in the 1960s that the department of Santa Cruz, together with the northeastern department of Beni, took off as the centre of the modern cocaine-manufacturing industry. The industry was run by two main groups: large cattle-ranchers in the Beni and the agro-business élite around Santa Cruz. Both had helped shape, and had benefited from, the Bolivian government's rural modernisation policies in the decades after the 1952 revolution, which tried to diversify production and exports to improve Bolivia's balance of trade. They had profited too from huge infusions of economic aid poured into Bolivia by the US during the dictatorship of General Banzer in the 1970s to contain the 'communist' threat.

With the agriculture boom of the 1960s and 1970s, farms and agro-businesses producing cotton, soya and cattle thrived. Their newly rich owners set up banks, import houses, car dealerships and money exchange houses, taking advantage of the favourable export, credit, and marketing policies introduced by the government. Santa Cruz estate owners were meanwhile gaining valuable experience in exporting commodities.

Then, in 1975, the cotton price collapsed. Members of the Cotton Growers' Association in Santa Cruz were given millions of dollars in credit as 'compensation'. In reality the money tended to be repayment for past political favours. Supervision of the 'loans' (which were never repaid) was minimal. Recipients used the money to buy large estates and town houses. Some also used it to lay the foundations of Bolivia's cocaine industry, building clandestine airstrips, and buying private planes and well armed bodyguards. To export cocaine, they used the routes they had used for decades to smuggle rubber to Argentina and whisky from Paraguay.

Bolivia's cocaine production began to catch up with that of Colombia and exports of cocaine soon exceeded all the country's legal exports. Alongside the country's traditional bourgeoisie a new class had sprung up: the narco-bourgeoisie.

The Beni cattle ranchers had also received preferential treatment from the government, including scarce financial and technical resources. They got support too from high-ranking military officers who had been given land concessions in the Beni region during the 1970s, often in return for political favours. Like the estate owners, the ranchers benefited from the fact that the vast Santa Cruz and Beni regions had always been areas over which the central government had little or no control.

A third group which helped set up the cocaine industry was the military, whose role will be examined in Chapter 5. Having been all but abolished in the 1952 revolution, the military establishment had regained much of its strength by the early 1960s, partly as a result of massive US aid. Under the dictatorship of General Banzer, government officials turned a blind eye to dabbling by the military in cocaine trafficking. Then, in 1980, a portly general called García Meza launched the most vicious coup in Bolivia's troubled history. Under García Meza and his Interior Minister Arce Gómez, dubbed the 'Minister of Cocaine', the right-wing faction of the military and the traffickers became one and the same thing.

BOLIVIA'S multimillion dollar cocaine industry is run by around 35 organisations, most of them family businesses centred around a single father figure with cousins, brothers, offspring and chums all giving a hand. Many of the top druglords are related by blood or intermarriage. They work separately, but share chemists, pilots, labs, assassins and government contacts when necessary. 'They are very smart at working together,' says a DEA source. 'If one trafficker suddenly gets an order from Colombia which he can't meet on his own, he rings a cousin and asks him to help out.' To export cocaine, the traffickers group in loosely organised cartels based in the Beni, Santa Cruz and Cochabamba, which are subdivided into smaller Mafias in Beni towns like Santa Ana de Yacuma, Riberalta and Guayaramerín.

The old breed were cocaine cowboys who donned dark glasses and gold chains, owned more houses than they could count, and swaggered about town with the confidence of men who knew they ran the place. They spurned Bolivian beer for imported British whisky, threw raucous parties and settled scores with impulsive savagery. In their local communities they played the role of feudal lord, befriending the rich, cheering the poor and acting the godfather at weddings and baptisms.

In one respect, though, they were totally different from their Colombian colleagues: whenever possible, they avoided violence. This was partly because as a country Bolivia, despite its history of coups, is far more pacific than Colombia. Also, murdering journalists, justice ministers, or innocent bystanders was not good for business. It merely drew unwelcome attention to their existence, especially from the *gringos*, and prompted massive reprisals from the army, police and DEA. The Bolivians were just as ruthless when it came to settling scores with other traffickers or informants, but as professionals, they made sure it was always done out of the public eye.

In the 1980s, the biggest *narco* was Roberto Suárez, now locked up in La Paz. Like many of his companions he began life as a cattle rancher who found that his remote jungle *haciendas* made ideal places in which to refine cocaine away from the eye of the authorities.

He was later supplanted by his nephew, Jorge Roca Suárez, who worked under the *nom de guerre* of Techo de Paja, on account of his blond hair. He was brought up in Los Angeles and spoke English like a *gringo*, but in 1981 he went to Bolivia to work for his uncle as a paste buyer. Having picked up the trade he set up a family business known as Los Techos and proceeded to undercut Suárez by selling to the Colombians at rock bottom prices.

With some of his family still in Florida, Techo had the ideal contacts to run an international trafficking business. He established routes to the US through Colombia, Mexico, and Panama. All his relatives worked for the family business. His brothers Felipe, Fernando and Oscar, bought the cocaine paste from the Chapare and transported it to labs in the Beni, helped by Techo's sisters Tita and Asunta. Blanca, his mother, collected dollar payments and sent them back to Bolivia. Soon Techo was turning over $10 million a year. He fronted it by buying mansions in Santa Cruz and a supermarket called Number One, which he registered in his sister's name. For the DEA and the Bolivian police, Techo was Bolivia's Number One *narco*.

In the mid-1980s, he set up business in Santa Ana de Yacuma, a dusty Wild West town in the Beni, an hour's flight north of Trinidad, the capital, and 130 miles from the Brazilian border. The only access to the town was by air, so Techo knew that if the authorities came looking for him he would hear about it long before they arrived. He built a 20-room mansion overlooking the central square and with a handful of other traffickers, including Suárez, set up what would become known as the Santa Ana cartel, or La Corporación.

Santa Ana's *narcos* were protected by heavily armed bodyguards (often Colombians) and the town's 16,000-odd inhabitants who knew they had little choice but to work for them. They knew that if they did not people would suspect them of being informants, and in any case there was little other employment. The town ran on cocaine, dumped and collected by small planes which buzzed in and out of its airstrip. The traffickers armed the locals with automatic weapons, turning Santa Ana into a place no policeman or DEA agent dared to go. Unclaimed bodies would sometimes be found rotting in the ditches around the town.

Like Suárez, Techo had good connections in the government. They were not connections you could pin down, of course. In 1988 a newspaper claimed to have spotted him at a party with Jaime Paz Zamora, later Bolivia's president, an allegation Paz denied. In 1986 he used his contacts to avoid being sentenced after police captured him in the Beni.

In the US, though, Techo did not have as many contacts. In December 1990 he was arrested by the US authorities while strolling on the outskirts of Los Angeles. Six months later his mother, brother and sister were picked up in Santa Cruz. Journalists were shown around his Santa Ana and Santa Cruz mansions, which the police had seized and which were to be turned into shelters for street children. By the time the children were due to move in, though, the houses were bare. The police who had captured them had gone on a rampage of looting. They had wrenched out the hand basins from the bathrooms, hi-fi systems from the living rooms, even the air-conditioning. Hair dryers and videos had mysteriously disappeared from the shelves of Number One, leaving a few rows of detergent and ketchup.

Meanwhile, a new, more sophisticated breed of traffickers was appearing. They still bought mansions and BMWs, but they learnt to be more discreet, which was necessary to avoid the attention of the US and Bolivian governments who were waking up to the fact that they had a 'cocaine problem'. Most, like Hugo Rivero Villavicencio, currently Bolivia's largest trafficker, prefer the seclusion of their Beni ranches or Santa Ana to the cities. When he stops in town he never spends more than three nights in the same house.

Rivero has had some nasty experiences. In 1987 the police raided his lakeside ranch, Primavera (Spring), which is an hour's flight north of Trinidad. The ranch, enclosed by a high white wall and equipped with its own airstrip, was as luxurious as any in Texas. In the front was an open-air thatched bar where guests sipped whiskies as they discussed deals or watched the sun set over the lake. Even the bodyguards' beds were carved from best Beni mahogany, and outside pure-bred stallions grazed in the paddocks. In the living room hung a stuffed bull's head, a symbol of the owner's *macho* prowess. Some 500 metres south of the house was a laboratory capable of making thousands of kilos of cocaine a week. The police turned it into a base and fuel depot for the Huey helicopters based in the town of Trinidad, thus enabling them to extend their range when raiding labs by another 100 miles.

Today the bar crawls with ants, and rags of dried beef hang from the washing line. In the living room, though, a few reminders of the former owner remain. The bull's head still hangs, 'it was too heavy to get down' explains one policeman, and a blown-up photograph of Rivero's eight year-old daughter in a yellow T-shirt still smiles down at the mansion's new inhabitants.

Rivero moved to Santa Ana, whose role as a drug trafficking centre had given it a reputation as the Medellín of Bolivia. At least 30 druglords had their homes here, some as big as palaces with solid gold taps. The *narcos* dispensed largesse like village squires, installing street lighting, erecting clinics and even building a *Casa de Cultura* with 5,000 books. Rivero, who was a sociable type, gave sumptuous parties and was well liked. In 1989 he was the target of a major night-time assault on Santa Ana by joint DEA and Bolivian police forces, but the whole town, including Rivero's bodyguards, rose in armed resistance, prompting a shootout in which four people were killed. Rivero, who had been tipped off about the raid several hours earlier, was nowhere to be found. Then, one day in 1990, he reportedly hit a journalist and was kicked out of town. He moved to Guayaramerín, a small town on the banks of the Mamoré, a tributary of the Amazon which runs through the Beni, where, at the time of writing, he still is.

Then there was Carmelo 'Meco' Domínguez, a quiet man in his mid-30s who worked with seven other groups to run one of Bolivia's biggest mafias. He had a paste-buying operation in the Chapare called Los Huatos, and big labs in the Beni. When police seized him and his assets in 1990 they found notebooks which showed he had export routes through Colombia, Mexico and bank accounts in Switzerland, Panama and the Bahamas. Meco was sent to San Pedro, but caused a rumpus when a few months later he paid his way out. Under US pressure he was hastily recaptured.

Others, like 'Lieutenant' Erwin Guzmán, and 'Captain' Jorge Flores, used to serve in the armed forces. 'Lieutenant' Guzmán retired from the air force 20 years ago but made good use of his experience in flying small planes. One of the longest established traffickers, he is believed to control most of the Chapare cocaine paste production, and has direct links with Medellín in Colombia. He is also one of the richest, estimated to make between $10 and $20 million a month. Like Rivero he lives in Santa Ana but never sleeps more than four nights in one place. He is careful not to flaunt his wealth. 'Guzmán likes to think of himself as a respectable *señor*,' says a police officer. 'He is one of the most intelligent traffickers, and is very legalistic.'

In July 1991 Guzmán and two other of Bolivia's 'top five', Winston Rodríguez and Antonio Nacif, turned themselves in in response to a government amnesty which promised no extradition to the US and reduced gaol terms to traffickers who surrendered of their own free will and confessed to their crimes within 120 days. In November, just before the deadline expired, Flores followed suit and gave himself up in Santa Cruz.

There are plenty more to fill their shoes, like Bismarck Barrientos, a former police officer who was thrown out of the police and set up as a narco-lawyer in Cochabamba. He has a reputation as a loud mouth and is one of the least liked traffickers. He owns Cochabamba's flashiest discotheque, *Reflejos* (Reflections), and several hotels. There are the Chávez brothers from Santa Cruz, nicknamed *Los Martillos* (The Hammers) because of their taste for violence. They are related by marriage to the Gasser family, one of Santa Cruz's oldest sugar oligarchy families, which later dabbled in cocaine. Then there is Isaac Chavarría, who was photographed escorting the president around the country during the 1988 election campaign and Oscar Roca, Techo's brother, who works as a pop singer in Santa Ana. And others whose names no-one yet knows.

WHILE Santa Cruz is the business headquarters of the cocaine industry, the Beni, a vast region of dusty tropical plains, meandering rivers and alligator-infested swamps a few hours to the northeast by plane, is where the cocaine is made. Stretching from the Andes to the Brazilian border, the Beni department covers 214,000 square kilometres, an area almost as big as Great Britain or Kansas.

In laboratories hidden under the thick jungle canopy, the next step of the cocaine-manufacturing process is carried out: the transformation of coca paste into cocaine sulphate, or base, and sometimes the final stage too, the turning of base into cocaine hydrochloride, or pure cocaine. Unlike the primitive 'mom and pop' paste pits of the Chapare, the Beni labs are sophisticated affairs which can cost from $500,000 to $1 million to set up.

The paste (or sometimes base too) is collected from the Chapare in light planes by paste buyers who work freelance or for a specific Mafia. It has to be done quickly to prevent the paste rotting in the Chapare's hot climate. A trafficker called Roberto describes how he picks up the paste from the Chapare:

> We leave Santa Cruz in the Cessna at 5.30 or 6.00 in the morning to arrive well before the police are up. There are usually four of us: a pilot, a controller (that's me), an analyst and an accountant. The flight to the Chapare takes about an hour. On the way we radio the intermediary on the ground to tell him we are coming and to check all's clear. If he says the police are around, we don't go. If it's OK he lays sheets on a stretch of road to make it smooth for us to land on, preferably a stretch with houses on either side, and fires shots in the air. These mean, 'The boss wants to buy, there's money to be paid.' Everybody sets out by car or on foot with whatever dope they have, maybe one kilo, maybe two or three. Once we've received the all-clear we land and go up a track just inside the jungle where everyone is waiting for us. Our analyst weighs the drugs on scales and checks their quality and weight; sometimes they cheat us and mix it with flour. On average we pay about $200 a kilo, although the price varies according to the competition. If there are a lot of traffickers wanting paste, the villagers ask for more. The analyst asks them if the dope is wet or dry. If it's wet, he 'punishes' the price. The trafficker doesn't like buying the paste wet because he doesn't have time to dry it and it's heavy, and he wants to get as much paste as he can onto the plane. The maximum load is 450 kilos. The accountant hands over a suitcase of

money, anything from $100,000 to $500,000, and the rest of us load the dope aboard. Not a second is lost. In fact it's done so fast that the pilot doesn't even turn off the engine. The whole process takes no more than four minutes.

The big traffickers bring bodyguards with them. The number of bodyguards varies according to who he is; some have as many as eight, partly as a status symbol. We don't usually bother. We just pay the police $10,000 a flight through our intermediary. We also pay the coca unions about $120 for them to use on public works. That way we keep the villagers happy and make sure they won't report on us.

It's another hour to the Beni. We radio to tell them we're coming and they clear the strip of metal barrels which we put to stop other planes landing, including police planes. The workers at the camp unload the *merca* as quickly as possible and take it to a spot one or two kilometres into the forest where it's processed. We take off again as soon as possible back to Santa Cruz; a plane on the strip is dangerously visible. If, for some reason we arrive late at night and can't take off, we cover the plane with leaves and branches to make it invisible, and stay the night.

Lab sites are chosen so as to be well outside the range of the Huey helicopters used by Bolivian and US law enforcement agents. Hidden under the trees, the labs are invisible from the air. Usually the only giveaway sign is a strip of pale green canvas carved out of the trees: the airstrip. 'You look for airstrips which don't seem to be attached to a ranch, and you can be sure it's a lab,' says a DEA agent. Traditionally, labs were semi-permanent installations which took a couple of months to construct, but as law enforcement efforts have been stepped up, traffickers have turned to mobile labs which can be quickly dismantled or moved on wheels.

The lab and living quarters are usually a few hundred yards from the strip, sometimes as far as a mile, so that if the police arrive there is still time to escape. Now, DEA sources say, labs are being built several miles from the strip and from there can only be reached by river, making them virtually impossible for outsiders to find. Cocaine is never kept on site, in case the lab is raided. It is hidden in stashes deep in the jungle. 'The DEA have never found our lab,' says Roberto. 'We see their helicopters flying over sometimes and have a good laugh.'

The camp is a self-contained community of anything from five to 50 workers, complete with laboratories, sleeping quarters, kitchens and latrines. Some even have gymnasiums, televisions and refrigerators, run on generators. Chemists, lab technicians, cooks and plane mechanics of all nationalities are flung together, bound by a common desire to make quick money. The chemists, known as 'cooks', tend to be Colombians, sent by the Colombian cartels to ensure the cocaine is of high quality. Some even have a Ph.D. 'They keep their recipes a closely guarded secret,' says Roberto. There tends to be bitter rivalry between the Colombians and Bolivians so Roberto keeps himself to himself. His favourite pastime is reading.

For security, lab employees are assigned one particular task, and are told only the name (or nickname) of the person directly above them. They know nothing about the operation as a whole or the name of the boss at the top. That way if anyone is caught, the others cannot talk.

The processes to make base and hydrochloride are similar to those to make paste. Two and a half kilos of paste are required to make one kilo of base, while just over a kilo of base makes a kilo of pure cocaine. A police officer described the process:

> When the traffickers are going to make base they say *Vamos a batir* (let's beat). They put the wet paste in a plastic bowl and in another they mix water and dilute sulphuric acid. They pour the acid into the first bowl and beat the mixture with a stick for about an hour until it turns a leaden grey. Then they add a solution of potassium permanganate which makes it turn a deep purple. Next they add some ammonia which precipitates what is now cocaine base. The chemist filters and washes it, then spreads it out to dry in the sun.
>
> The next stage, making the finished cocaine, is a bit more complicated. They put the base in a container, pour on some ether to dissolve it, then filter the mixture. Next they add hydrochloric acid mixed with acetone. The proportions have to be exactly right, a quarter of a litre of acid to a kilo of paste. They mix it thoroughly. The cocaine begins to precipitate out and the mixture turns yellow and gives off a strong smell like a chemist shop.
>
> Next they add ether, just a tiny bit, and again being careful to get the proportions exactly right. They have to be careful that there are no naked flames, as ether is highly inflammable. Some chemists have been burned after ether caught alight and exploded in their faces. They wait two or three hours while the mixture turns white and the cocaine solidifies into tiny crystals. The mixture is filtered and the cocaine spread out on big gauze trays on a metal table and dried under strong gas or electric-powered lamps suspended above. The cook has to be quick in case a wind gets up and blows dirt onto the cocaine. The drying takes between two hours and half a day.
>
> When the dope is perfectly dry, it's put on tin foil and compressed by a machine into one kilogram bricks, just as if it was sweets or cheeses. The trafficker then stamps his trademark on, to show that it is his. They don't put a name of course. Instead it's a symbol, like a moon with a cross beside it, which people in the trade recognise. The bricks are then wrapped in brown paper and packed in bundles of 100 ready to be loaded into the plane.

The Bolivians leave it to others to fly the cocaine to Colombia for further processing if it is base, or to distribution points in Colombia or elsewhere in South America or the Caribbean if it is finished cocaine. Around 90 per cent of Bolivian base is sold to Colombians who know the ropes and have the contacts with the US. The arrangement suits (or did until recently) the peace-loving Bolivians who feel like fish out of water outside their country and like to avoid the hassles and rip-offs that go with distribution. The Colombians radio the lab to say what day and time they are coming, and fly in via Brazil. They arrive with large plastic bags crammed with dollar notes (the Bolivians insist on small denominations in case they are faked) which they exchange for cocaine.

Like any multinational business, the cocaine industry has a complex infrastructure. People must be employed, for example, to smuggle in chemicals from Europe, the US or other South American countries. Sulphuric acid and potassium permanganate are brought by road or river from Brazil, with payoffs made to customs officials on the border. Ammonia and acetone are sent from Chile and Argentina. The quantities of 'precursor' chemicals used by the industry are staggering. Some labs have been found with as many as ten 200-litre barrels of ether, worth a total of $50,000. One laboratory had 600. Destruction of the chemicals can seriously dent a trafficker's operations. But the traffickers are several steps ahead: they are now reported to be recycling chemicals to avoid the risk and cost of importing them. 'The traffickers have become very environmentally aware,' says an Interpol agent sarcastically. 'They're heavily into recycling.'

Equipment is needed too, like powerful lamps and straining and drying tables, propane fuel tanks, water pumps and generators to provide power for cooking and hot water. These are smuggled by air from cities like Santa Cruz or Cochabamba or by land from Brazil. Traffickers also need transport; they buy Cessna 206s from Santa Cruz or Miami for about $60,000 a piece, removing identity plates to make it more difficult for police to trace them. Others steal their planes from remote ranches in Brazil, Peru or Bolivia, confident that owners will not risk their lives by reporting the incident. Weapons, used by the bodyguards to defend the labs, are imported through Colombia from the US or Europe. The most common are Israeli-made Uzis, Belgian FALNs and Russian AK-47s, but US-made assault rifles have also been found.

Security is backed up by a complex intelligence network made up of scores of radio operators and look-outs posted in the jungle and in cities like Santa Cruz and Cochabamba. Regular payments are made to the police in return for tip-offs about raids. Informants are used to misinform the DEA or the Bolivian narcotics police. An informant, for instance, tips them off about a laboratory which is no longer in use. While they are distracted in searching for the lab, the trafficker continues operations unhindered. The traffickers can afford to pay well. As one UMOPAR officer says, 'We pay informants well, but the traffickers pay even better.' People who inform on the *narcos*, on the other hand, are dealt with by hired assassins who hack them to bits.

IN THE late 1980s, Bolivia's cocaine industry underwent a major change. The Bolivians had traditionally sold their cocaine to Colombians, but often never got paid, because the Colombians only handed over the dollars if they got their loads to the US. At other times the Colombians never turned up to pick up the shipments they had ordered. The Bolivians lost millions. 'The Colombians think they own us,' complained one trafficker. 'They pay what they want and then over-charge the Americans.'[1] A peaceful people, they also found the Colombians' Hollywood-gangster style of doing business distasteful. They turned to other nationalities as middlemen and insisted on 'money up front' arrangements.

Instead of going via Colombia and from there to the US, cocaine began to take new routes through countries like Brazil, Argentina, Paraguay and Chile. Quietly, the Chilean port of Iquique, and the Argentine capital Buenos Aires, turned into distribution centres almost as important as Medellín and Cali in Colombia. Seizures in Brazil, where Rio de Janeiro has become a major transhipment port, doubled from 1989 to 1990 and continue to soar. Some cocaine went to supply a growing local appetite. The rest went to the US or, increasingly, to Europe, Africa and even Japan, where prices were far higher. While the Colombians tend to target Spain, the Bolivians' preferred European destinations are Britain, France and Italy.

The other change was that the Bolivians were no longer willing to be poorly paid suppliers of coca paste or base while their Colombian counterparts, who refined it into hydrochloride, raked in the profits. They decided to increase their profits by doing all the refining themselves. They set up their own hydrochloride laboratories, and left paste-making (and sometimes base) to peasants in the Chapare. The mark-ups are dramatic: by selling paste, a trafficker gets only $250 a kilo. With base he can earn six or seven times that amount. With hydrochloride, the profits are even greater, selling at between $1,600 and $2,500 a kilo. Bolivian labs are now among some of the biggest in South America, some worth up to $1 million, and capable of making up to 850 kilos. In 1987 a DEA informant reported seeing 17 landing fields with at least five tonnes of cocaine at each: a total of 100 and 5,000 kilos. He called it 'the General Motors of cocaine'.

The crack-down on drug mafias in Colombia in 1989 and 1990 speeded up the trend. Bolivian traffickers found they had no-one to buy their partly processed cocaine which was rapidly stockpiling and going mouldy in the humid jungle heat. They were forced to refine it themselves and to find other nationalities to distribute it. By 1990 one in four labs made hydrochloride. Bolivia exported an estimated 250-300 tonnes, making it the world's second largest producer of market-ready cocaine.

Some labs are now reportedly run by Colombians who had moved to Bolivia after being squeezed out of Colombia. It was not too difficult because over the years they had got to know the Bolivians well. Now, instead of simply acting as buyers, chemists and bodyguards, Colombians ran laboratories of their own. In August 1990, an ether condenser coil which recycles ether, previously seen only in Colombia, was found at a laboratory in the Beni. 'The traffickers get squeezed one place, they're going to look for another,' said Gonzálo Torrico, the under secretary for social defence in the Interior Ministry.[2]

With the entry of Colombians into Bolivia came fears they would bring with them their violent way of doing business. So far, reports vary. Some enforcement agents say they have noticed an increase in the number of automatic weapons pointed at them when they raid labs. Even at paste labs, bodyguards who would before never have been armed now carry 9mm machine guns. Others say they have yet to notice a real change.

THE traffickers' fantastic wealth enables them to infiltrate every state institution from the military, the police, the judiciary and the government, to the media and the Chapare coca farmers' federations. Bribes, in return for protection, are an integral part of traffickers' budgets, and have the important side-effect of undermining people's faith in the state and its institutions. Payments are made to local and district police chiefs to ensure they do not raid their labs, and tip them off when a raid is imminent. Airport and customs officials are befriended and paid off. If traffickers are unlucky enough to get arrested, they bribe judges or prison guards to get them out of gaol. They start by asking the guard for a weekend out, for which they pay around $300. Then they ask for a week at a time, which costs a bit more. Then one time they don't return. If the guards won't play ball, the trafficker works on his lawyer to arrange the tampering of the evidence. 'The trafficker's lawyer has a word with the police who say they will fiddle the evidence for a sum, say $50,000,' says an intelligence source. 'The lawyer tells the trafficker that the police want $100,000, which the trafficker hands over. That way both do well out it.'

According to Western intelligence sources, part of the payments made to the police filter up, via intermediaries, usually former police or military officers, to a few key government ministries, like the Ministry of the Interior. The money may be paid via holding companies or banks. Two trafficking groups reportedly make direct payments to top-level politicians, lessening the risk of being tripped up by the odd honest police officer. One druglord was estimated to be paying a high-level cabinet minister between $1 and $2 million a year. Usually, though, pressure is exerted on politicians in more subtle ways, like contributing to election campaigns, usually through front organisations, or providing planes or cars to ferry politicians around on the campaign trail. They make *regalos* (presents) of flashy cars, or houses.

Some barons have been so powerful they have been able to establish dialogues with governments. In June 1983 Roberto Suárez met President Siles Zuazo's narcotics adviser, Rafael Otazo, and offered the Bolivian government $2,000 million in four $500-million instalments. As a quid pro quo, Suárez wanted a free hand to run his trafficking operations in the Beni. Although Siles denied he had sent Otazo, the outcry over the affair nearly toppled his government.

Official support, however, is not enough to protect the traffickers. They depend on grassroots support too. They buy this in rural areas by acting as Robin Hood figures, providing services which the government cannot afford. They install street lighting, build schools and clinics, or confetti $10 bills to the poor. The cost to a trafficker of such charity is budgeted for as protection money.

The government, whose coffers are virtually empty, cannot compete. 'When we carry out raids, we give the people nothing, not even pencils or school-books,' says a frustrated UMOPAR commander.

> The *narco*, on the other hand, leaves things when he comes. People go to him and say 'We need a school' or 'My child is ill. Can you give me money to buy him some medicine?' and he gives them cash. The *narcos* haven't been to university but they are damned good at PR. When they go to a village they make a contribution to the local economy: they pay well for the hotel, they buy cigarettes, they eat in the local restaurant. So the people like them. Last month, a trafficker even paid for a live orchestra to play in Isinuta. He bought everybody beers. It must have cost him $200, but that's nothing for him.

The traffickers also manipulate public opinion through the media. US-financed anti-drugs campaigns are portrayed as attacks on Bolivian sovereignty and on the sanctity of the coca leaf. Traffickers are shown not as criminals but as respectable *señores*. The drug barons use the media to smear politicians, branding anyone they dislike, or who gets in their way, as a trafficker. Accusations like this become so commonplace that in the end no-one takes any notice.

Journalists who probe links between the traffickers and the government are intimidated or attacked. In 1987, a journalist on the Cochabamba newspaper *Los Tiempos*, was attacked in La Paz by paramilitary gunmen and had his passport and tape recorder stolen after he wrote an article about trafficking inside the Bolivian navy. In 1987 a member of the Canelas family, which owns *Los Tiempos*, was kidnapped, reportedly by a Brazilian group, and the family forced to pay a $100,000 ransom. 'After that the family told us not to publish things about the *narcos*. They didn't want any more problems,' says the journalist.

Sometimes the cocaine barons stand as political candidates or mayors or install a proxy candidate. More often though, they want to avoid being so prominent. Despite their ability to influence, cajole and threaten, most traffickers do not exert or aspire to political power. Perhaps they learnt their lesson from the 1980 military dictatorship of General García Meza, which brought the traffickers unwelcome exposure. 'After that traffickers saw they could live with democracy quite happily,' says Roger Cortez, Bolivia's best-known investigative journalist. 'They preferred to work through malleable politicians than to stand for office themselves.' Rather than political power, which would interfere with the work of running a business, traffickers seek protection of people, assets, transit routes and cash flows. Paradoxically, the traffickers are so powerful already they do not need political power.

* * *

INSIDE La Paz's San Pedro gaol, a prisoner paces up and down the length of his cell and draws on his Marlboro cigarette. The cell is no ordinary cell: about 12 by 14 feet, it is six times the size of most, and has a television and access to a telephone. In fact it is so luxurious compared to San Pedro's other hovels that they call it Hotel San Pedro. But then its inmate is no ordinary prisoner: he is Roberto Suárez, Bolivia's legendary King of Cocaine.

Dressed in white boots and trousers, he is waiting for me as I pay my way past the prison guards and slip through a large metal gate into his cell. His bumbling bonhomie, dapper looks and greased-back dyed brown hair give him an uncanny resemblance to Ronald Reagan. And like Reagan, Suárez is a fan of the former British prime minister. 'How's Margaret?' he quips, giving me a bear hug as affectionately as if he were my uncle.

He motions me to a table with a plastic table-cloth and pours me a Pepsi Cola in a disposable cup. I am seated next to a pretty Bolivian dolly bird who cannot be more than 20. The girl, presumably one of Suárez's retinue of female admirers, smiles a lot but says nothing. In the far corner of the room, Suárez's wife is crouched over a sewing machine, smoking. She too is silent.

Once the head of a multibillion empire that supplied Colombia's Medellín cartel with virtually all its paste and base, even in prison Suárez has the status of king. The guards respectfully address him as Don Roberto and smuggle him bottles of whisky. Deferential government officials regularly pop in to talk business. They slip in through a discreet private entrance in a quiet side street, out of sight of the queues of bowler-hatted Indian women jostling in front of the main gate. Suárez rarely mixes with the pitiful specimens of humanity in the main part of the prison, except to visit the clinic. 'It makes me too sad,' he says.

Suárez, like most big-time drug traffickers, lives in the exclusive part of San Pedro known as La Posta. There are about 40 druglords in at present, mostly Bolivians plus a few Colombians and Brazilians. They bring their bodyguards to protect themselves from each other and employ the guards to carry messages, run errands and tip them off when an unwelcome visitor has arrived. A few cells down from Suárez is 'Meco' Domínguez. He is so rich and influential he would not have stayed in more than a fortnight were it not for the watchful eye of the US embassy. None the less he is hardly treated like an ordinary prisoner: he managed to get a private telephone installed, which he used to continue business as usual. Dubbed the *narcoteléfono*, it was removed a few weeks later when the Americans got wind of it. Another theory held that the Americans themselves had installed it so that they could monitor 'Meco's' calls

Suarez's cell is lime green, but mouldy patches of damp are appearing on the ceiling. It is dimly lit and smells a little musty. Sentimental posters of white horses galloping through the sea at sunset and a European forest in autumn add superficial cheer. In the far corner stands a new white exercise bike and a collection of medicines which Suárez uses to treat his heart condition. There is a cooker, a refrigerator and a cupboard of rice and pasta, brought in by Suárez's wife.

Separated from the rest of the room by plywood cupboards and fading carnival decorations suspended from the ceiling are two beds. Over one is a list of the Ten Commandments and a picture of Jesus: 'I'm a devout Catholic. God is the only judge,' explains Suárez, 'but I don't bother with going to mass: priests are another of society's farces'. Slouched on the other bed, two tiny dark-haired figures watch comic strips on television. The boys, aged six and seven, are the youngest of Suárez's numerous offspring.

'The real king of cocaine,' says Suárez animatedly, 'is the US. But instead, they blame us. And they corrupt our children by putting awful adverts on television showing drug addicts looking like corpses. The other day my sons asked me "Daddy, what is dope?" "It's a kind of medicine," I told them.'

Nobody quite knows if Suárez's madcap tomfoolery is put on or a sign of his growing senility. But it's difficult not to smile at some of the more bizarre lines of the wily druglord's song. Take the mistaken identity line, for instance. With an air of almost total sincerity he explains: 'They were looking for a Roberto Suárez who was a drug trafficker, but they got the wrong one. In Bolivia there are 174 Roberto Suárez. My name is Roberto Suárez Gómez.'

Playing on his title as king is another favourite. 'They call me the king of cocaine but actually I'm the king of coca. I have always fought to keep the price of cocaine high to save my people and humanity from the brutal effects of trafficking. Now,' he adds, with unabashed self-importance, 'I am king of the fight against cocaine, the terrible scourge of our people which is poisoning our children.' He pauses for effect, then wags his finger like a school teacher. 'The only person who can save Bolivia is Roberto Suárez.' Anger takes over.

> It's a total farce my being in here. The government is using me as a scapegoat to convince the Americans that they're doing something against drug trafficking. While I've been stuck in this room for two years, traffickers in this prison are paying 2,000 bucks a week to walk free in the streets and carry on their business. The only ones left in here are traffickers who have gone bust and the wretched stompers. I'm being used to cover up their circus. It's like trying to blot out the

sun with one finger. If there were any justice in Bolivia I would have been let out long ago.

Suárez's most virulent anger is directed against the US. The reason the Americans are trying to destroy Bolivia's coca fields, he says, is because they want to control the cocaine industry themselves. He illustrates what he sees as the US attitude towards Bolivia with the story of how, in 1963, he visited the White House with his friend Frank Sinatra. 'I looked at the map on the wall,' he says, 'and Bolivia didn't even exist.'

The drugs trade will never disappear, he says, because both the US and the Bolivian government have too much to lose. 'Here the trafficker is the government, there it's the system. Everybody's in it, from the State Department to the CIA.'

US DEA agents first became aware of the name of Roberto Suárez in 1977 when informants said he was supplying huge amounts of cocaine base to customers in Mexico and Colombia who converted it into refined cocaine. In fact, Suárez had already been operating for years and he knew far more about the agents than they did about him. He had files, passed onto him by the interior ministry, on every agent, complete with photographs and personal histories.

Suárez was born in 1932 to one of Bolivia's oldest and most aristocratic families. His parents were educated in Europe (mainly Germany) and a distant relation had even worked as *chargé d'affaires* in London. Brought up on the family cattle ranches, Suárez learnt to ride a horse almost before he could walk. Later he divided his time between his various Beni *estancias*, his home town of Santa Ana, and his town houses in Santa Cruz. Don Roberto was a family man, much respected in the community. He had four children by his first wife — Heidi, Gary, Ana María and Robbie. Heidi was a stunner, who once became Miss Bolivia. But Suárez's favourite was Robbie, a reserved boy who mastered five languages, spoke with a Texan accent after a US education and had a passion for archaeology. Robbie had been trained as a pilot, so was useful to the operations of his father whom he idolised. 'He was crazy about Suárez,' recalls a former neighbour in Santa Cruz. 'He saw him as a god. He was perfect. He loved him too much.'

Suárez began to dabble in cocaine. During the dictatorship of General Banzer, a friend of his, Suárez knew the authorities would not trouble him on his remote Beni ranches. Suárez set up a small family business with a friend called Marcelo Ibáñez. Gradually it expanded and he linked up with other cattle ranchers who had also branched into cocaine and were setting up a cartel with its business headquarters in Santa Cruz. Soon they were exporting thousands of pounds of cocaine base to Colombia, where Suárez had contacts in the Medellín cartel. The Colombians sent their men to collect the cocaine and chemists to ensure he got his recipes right. Suárez was Bolivia's first big timer.

In Santa Ana, where Suárez lived as a feudal lord, he was known fondly as Don Roberto or El Padrino (The Godfather) or Papito (Daddy). He distributed crumbs of his wealth by restoring churches, building clinics and providing electricity with generators left over from his labs, luxuries which no government had ever provided. He even bought them a satellite dish, enabling the inhabitants to watch Mexican soap operas on television for the first time. In return, Suárez gained their allegiance and ensured they would keep quiet if the authorities came looking for him.

But cocaine was a risky business, and by 1979 Suárez was in serious financial difficulties. He applied for a loan in Bolivia but failed. Eventually he secured a $1 million loan from a finance company in New York. The only snag was that they wanted a commission of $250,000 and the money had to be collected from a sister bank in Monte Carlo. But Suárez badly needed it, so agreed.

After a while, though, he started having doubts, so went in person to Monte Carlo and hired a private detective, who discovered that the company did not exist. Suárez flew to Miami and filed a complaint with the FBI who told him the company was made up of professional swindlers.

'My father returned to Bolivia after this bad experience and used a little of his own money in the political campaign in favour of... [air force general] Juan Pereda,'[3] recalled Robbie later. 'After all this, since the financial situation was getting worse, my father decided to improve his financial situation by getting in to the cocaine traffic. At the time a lot of people in Bolivia were trading in cocaine.'[4] (Since Suárez's business had been going for years, Robbie's account is almost certainly disingenuous.)

Meanwhile, through Banzer, Suárez had made the acquaintance of another man of German descent called Klaus Barbie, once the head of the Gestapo in Lyons, who had been living in Bolivia since 1951 under the name of Klaus Altmann. Under Banzer, Barbie had worked for the Ministry of the Interior and for 'Department Seven' of the army in Cochabamba, which specialised in 'psychological operations'. Suárez found Barbie's violent ways distasteful, but recognised that his contacts in the underworld of crime and his intimate knowledge of Bolivia's security apparatus made him just the man to advise him on the delicate matter of protecting his drug runners from Colombian dealers, who were a constant threat. Barbie provided him with a 28 year-old 'minder' called Joachim Fiebelkorn. A colleague of Fiebelkorn's recalls how Barbie spotted him: 'Roberto Suárez was expanding his business and was having trouble with the Colombian dealers. He had plenty of men, but he needed someone he could trust to organise and train them and help him fight the Colombians. Klaus Altmann brought Joachim over from Paraguay to work for Suárez.'[5]

After lengthy negotiations, in late 1978, Suárez commissioned Barbie and Fiebelkorn to assemble a small but vicious army of Fascist bodyguards who, for substantial payments, would give him absolute loyalty. They called themselves the Fiancés of Death after a song that had been sung by the French Foreign Legion.

'During our time with Suárez,' recalled Fiebelkorn later, 'there was always trouble with the Colombians.' At one point, according to a former member of the group, they placed bazookas along the airstrip and fired at the Colombian dealers waiting to take delivery of the drug. 'We didn't have much trouble after that.'

The thugs also protected Suárez himself. 'He always had a guard of 10 or 15 people equipped with machine pistols,' said Fiebelkorn. 'Wherever he landed, there was an enormous reception, as if the president of Bolivia was arriving. I tramped along, immediately behind him, with my machine pistol.'[6]

Eventually Suárez decided the Colombians were causing so much trouble he would try to cut them out and deal directly with the US. His big chance came in May 1980 when a US dealer said he wanted to buy 500 kilos of cocaine base. In fact the dealer was a DEA agent, whose sting operation very nearly decapitated Suárez's network for ever.

The deal had been months in the planning. Earlier that year a DEA agent based in Buenos Aires called Mike Levine had met Marcelo Ibáñez, Suárez's trusted friend and business partner, in a nightclub overlooking the old port, La Boca. Levine convinced Ibáñez that his syndicate controlled clandestine airstrips and could manipulate customs and law enforcement agencies in Miami. Ibáñez assured him supply was no problem: he could provide 2,240 pounds of cocaine a month. Levine then invited Suárez and Ibáñez to come up to Miami to look over his set-up in Florida.

The DEA hired a lavish beach-side mansion in Fort Lauderdale, a dummy laboratory manned by a DEA chemist and three suitcases crammed with $9 million worth of notes. The DEA's most attractive female agents were seconded to the house as maids and escorts for the Bolivians. Another undercover agent, Richard Fiano, acted as chauffeur and boss of the Florida part of the operation. Enticing Suárez to Florida, however, proved more difficult than Levine had anticipated. Only Ibáñez turned up, and he insisted the Americans go to the Bolivians not the other way round. Levine was forced to agree. The Americans would fly to Bolivia to collect 500 kilos of cocaine base for which they would pay $8.5 million. Half the money would be paid as the plane left Bolivia, the rest when it landed in Miami.

On 16 May Fiano, three pilots and Ibáñez set out in a rusty Corvair 240 from Fort Lauderdale, Florida.[7] It took them several days to get to Bolivia because the plane broke down and had to be repaired *en route*. At Manaus, their final refuelling point, the party met Techo de Paja, Suárez's young nephew, who gave them maps and instructions on how to find the landing strip, near Lake Rogagua in the Beni. To Fiano's disappointment, Suárez was not there. He had sent Robbie instead. After an hour a Cessna arrived with the 854 pounds of cocaine base wrapped in bin liners. Robbie supervised workers who loaded the base plus a couple of pounds of hydrochloride as a sample of goodwill. Robbie and Ibáñez chatted as a DEA pilot took photographs.

'I looked through about 1,700 kilos of cocaine to find you the best,' Robbie said. 'If everything goes according to plan we'll be able to deliver the rest later.' The overloaded plane took off, only just managing to avoid crashing into the lake. Fiano radioed Levine in Miami to tell him the deal had been done. Ibáñez radioed his contact in Miami whom Suárez had chosen to collect the $9 million.

His name was Alfredo 'Cutuchi' Gutiérrez. He ran an air taxi business in Santa Cruz and had previously been president of the Santa Cruz Chamber of Commerce. He was to pick up the money from a DEA agent called José Hinojosa whom he knew as Pepe. Gutiérrez, Suárez had assured Pepe on the phone, was a man of utmost confidence and had collected money for him five times before. He was paying him $50,000 to pick up $4.25 million and deliver it to Bolivia. After that he was to fly back to Miami to pick up the rest of the money. Just in case, Suárez sent a 'minder' for Gutiérrez, called Roberto Gasser, a member of the Santa Cruz sugar oligarchy family.

At 11.00 a.m. on 22 May Pepe rang Gutiérrez who was staying at the Everglades Hotel in Miami and told him to sit tight until given instructions. He gave Gutiérrez a number to call if necessary and said he would ring again later. That evening Gutiérrez rang Pepe to see if the money could be paid as a cashier's cheque rather than cash. Pepe said he was sorry but he could only give cash. Just before midnight, Gutiérrez rang him to check what denomination bills they would be. They would be large bills, replied Pepe wearily. Gutiérrez was pleased: he didn't like small bills.

The next morning, at 11.15, Pepe rang Suárez senior, who said the aircraft had departed at 10.45. He requested the money be transferred quickly as it was Friday and he was afraid the vault would be closing. Two hours later, Pepe was ready. He called Gutiérrez to say he would pick him up at the Everglades Hotel with an associate (Levine). Gutiérrez recognised Pepe immediately and introduced himself as Alfredo. The four climbed into a hired car and drove to the Commercial Bank of Kendall on Miami's South Dixie Highway.

Fidgeting nervously, Gutiérrez was eager to chat.

'How's the plane going?' he asked Pepe.

'It's due in Miami tomorrow afternoon,' replied Pepe, who was recording Gutiérrez's every word.

'You know, I don't think we should use Corvairs any more. They're too large, they attract too much goddamned attention. In future we should use Merlins. They're much less obvious. And you can use modern communications systems like you use in homes and boats, to avoid them eavesdropping on you.'

The men fell silent for a moment. Gutiérrez asked if they had bought any hydrochloride from Suárez. He praised Suárez's manufacturing and distribution operation, which he claimed made almost daily deliveries to the Colombians. It ran 'smooth as silk', he said.

At the bank, the men entered a private cubicle in the safety deposit box area. One agent obtained three boxes which contained $2.2 million, $2 million and $300,000 respectively. One box also contained half a pound of cocaine as a sample. Gutiérrez fingered it. It wasn't as good as his product, he said. His was rockier, which meant higher strength and purity. The men secured the safety deposit boxes and gave Gutiérrez a fake key. They left the bank.

On the way back to the Everglades, Gutiérrez seemed relaxed. In Bolivia, he said, Suárez and his organisation were the powers that counted. In Santa Cruz, Suárez dictated who was arrested and who was left alone. No cocaine entered or left Bolivia without Suárez knowing about it.

'Why don't your people consider buying an island off the coast of Panama or Venezuela?' Gutiérrez asked. 'You'd have total security. With yachts and aircraft you could deliver up to 2,000 kilos of cocaine off Florida.' Pepe and his friend said it was a good idea and they would think about it. 'By the way,' Gutiérrez said, 'could you let me out at the Dupont Plaza?'

Gutiérrez got out at the hotel where he had arranged to meet Gasser. Gasser had been chosen to transport the money to Bolivia because he had political contacts which would enable him to avoid having to declare it. A while later, the two men returned to the Commercial Bank of Kendall. Gutiérrez signed a visitation slip to see the safety deposit boxes. The two were immediately arrested.

In gaol, Gutiérrez asked to speak to a DEA agent about his involvement in the deal. They talked. Gutiérrez agreed to call Roberto Suárez in Santa Cruz to tell him that he had the money and that everything was going smoothly. The agent listened to the conversation between Suárez and Gutiérrez.

'I want you to return to Bolivia immediately with the money,' said Suárez. 'Then I want you to go back to Florida next week. The money should be $4,250,000. I want it before the end of the day.' Suárez told Gutiérrez to stay on the phone as the 'boss', a man called Marcelo, wanted to speak to him. 'I don't want any excuses,' Marcelo yelled. 'Just bring the money to Santa Cruz. I don't want any more phone calls.' He hung up.

Gutiérrez was taken to Dade County Jail, while Gasser rang Suárez to tell him that he and Gutiérrez were under arrest and the money would not be reaching Bolivia. No formal charges were made against Gasser who returned to Bolivia the same day, but Gutiérrez was indicted on charges of

conspiring to smuggle cocaine into the US and distribute it. On 3 June a
Federal Grand Jury returned indictments against Suárez, his son and Ibáñez,
as well as Gutiérrez.

Bail for Gutiérrez was set at $3 million in cash but was later lowered by
the Miami judge to $1 million after he had received affidavits from Bolivia.
Gutiérrez quickly collected the money together and caught the next plane
home to Bolivia. Back home Gutiérrez and Suárez put a $200,000 price tag
on Levine's head. 'Amazingly, the biggest sting operation in law-enforce-
ment history was suddenly without any defendants,' said Levine later. Not
until he discovered that Suárez, with the help of the CIA, was in the meantime funding a coup to oust the elements in the Bolivian government who
had cooperated with the sting, did Levine believe he knew why.[8]

Meanwhile the uncertainty which had racked Bolivia since Banzer had
been deposed was worrying Suárez and his colleagues who saw it as a threat
to their operations. They decided to install a government of their own. In
July 1980, a right-wing military government, led by General García Meza,
seized power. US intelligence reports suggested that Suárez and Barbie had
taken a large part in planning and funding the takeover.

The next 13 months were paradise for Suárez, who built up his empire
into a multimillion dollar business. He profited from an arrangement set up
by the Interior Minister, Colonel Arce Gómez, whereby cocaine seized from
traffickers who were not paying protection was delivered to traffickers who
were. 'It is impossible to calculate the money [the drug barons] made,' said
an analyst at the time. 'Think of a preposterous figure, double it and know
damned well that you've made a gross underestimate.'[9]

Suárez kept much of his money in Switzerland, and sent various
members of his family to keep an eye on it. In December 1981 Robbie, now
22, went there 'to study', staying with a family friend called Giancarlo Pace
in a small village outside Locarno where his brother had already been living
for some time. He got there from Madrid using a forged Colombian passport.

With him Robbie brought $250,000 which he claimed was to pay for a
Porsche and a Mercedes he had bought, but was actually mostly money his
father wanted put away in a Swiss Bank. Robbie's mother, who was also
living in Switzerland, had ten cheques with a total value of $100,000. 'I
knew it was dirty money, product of cocaine trafficking because my father
told me himself,' Robbie later told an interrogator. 'My father told me he had
amassed $500,000... from... cocaine and that he was going to use it for the
family. He was afraid for his life, the police were looking for him and he
wanted this money to be in a safe place in case something should happen to
him.'[10]

Swiss police in Berne were watching Robbie carefully after receiving a
telex from the DEA in Buenos Aires in early 1980. At 7.00 a.m. one day in
January 1982 they struck.

One of the six police officers who arrested him recalls the event.

> I personally rang the door bell many times. No-one answered. I... gave the order to force in the door. We entered the building which was a large home.... We split up in order to search different rooms. I went into a room with a female agent, where the sister of Roberto Suárez, [Heidi], slept. Then two or three... of my... colleagues went into another room where they found Roberto Suárez Junior who was with someone else... a Bolivian... Ovando Luis Landívar.'

Robbie's account was different.[11]

> I was sleeping. We were in an apartment of a friend of mine's... and all I remember is when I woke up there was a uniformed policeman... beating my face and he had his knee on top of my chest. I didn't know what was happening. I started screaming and I was begging him to stop 'Please stop, stop'. I was knocked down from the bed... to the floor. They just kept beating me, then another two policemen... started beating me with their rifle butts. I was crying.

Robbie was imprisoned, then in August transferred to solitary confinement in another gaol. 'I didn't eat as my mouth was swollen and I was very sick,' he recalled later. 'I asked for a lawyer. One prosecutor said 'Traffickers in Switzerland die before they get a lawyer.'

> At 3.30 [one morning] I asked 'Where are you taking me.' They said they didn't know. I said I want to see a lawyer. I grabbed a fork that I had with my food that I had eaten the night before, and I put it to my throat and told them I would kill myself if they didn't take me to a lawyer. One man in the cell hit me on the back of the head and I lost consciousness. When I woke up I was handcuffed in a van, and I was on a road somewhere. I was at the airport. They put me in the cell and two men came in and said 'We are US marshals, and you are now under arrest.'

Robbie was flown to the US and on the way, according to his lawyer, was 'repeatedly threatened with his life'. At the airport, his old 'friend' DEA agent Rickey Fiano, was waiting for him.

Suárez Senior was furious. According to internal DEA files, Suárez hired eight mercenaries to kidnap two federal judges in Miami. In desperation he wrote to President Reagan and offered to turn himself in if in return the US wrote off Bolivia's foreign debt and released his son. Surprisingly, Reagan did not respond. But Robbie was acquitted anyway after a Miami jury believed his word over those of four DEA agents, a fact that was to gall the DEA for years afterwards.

In the meantime, Suárez had woven a network of connections that stretched from the Amazon to Guadalajara, from Miami to Spain. He relied on a group of young Bolivians, including his nephew Techo de Paja, to buy paste from smaller producers and get it to transhipment points. When it came to exporting cocaine, his most important contact was a man called Pablo Escobar, who headed Colombia's Medellín cartel. Suárez became one of the cartel's largest base suppliers. In 1984 when the Colombian National Police raided a vast cocaine processing complex owned by the Medellín cartel known as Tranquilandia, a ledger showed that Suárez had supplied 700 kilos of paste.

Suárez became so rich, legend had it that like Midas everything he touched turned to gold. His massive fortune bought guns, protection and power over provincial and even central government. He owned over 500,000 hectares of land and more cattle ranches than he could count. It was said he had as many mistresses as ranches. Protected by platoons of paramilitary mercenaries, and constantly on the move, Suárez eluded any police he had not managed to pay off. This was the heyday of the reign of the King of Cocaine.

In 1983 Suárez flew a group of journalists to visit him at his largest ranch, Quemalia. He met them with a baby leopard in his arms, and went on to brag that he had a fortune of $400 million 'which had nothing to do with drug trafficking' and a fleet of '40 planes, all of them modern' (although no-one ever saw them).

Suárez was seemingly untouchable. Even the Americans could not get him. Suárez laughed when he heard in April 1983 that a federal jury in Miami had indicted Arce Gómez and six other Bolivian officials for conspiring with him and nine other druglords to export cocaine to the US. A few months later when the interior minister sent troops into the Beni looking for Suárez, the druglord took out newspaper ads accusing the minister of being a trafficker himself.

But the king's good fortune could not last for ever. In 1984, the Colombians, who had been paying him $14,000 a kilo for coca paste, dropped the price to $9,000. Suárez refused to sell, insisting on the higher price.

It cost Suárez his supremacy. While Suárez stockpiled his cocaine, Techo agreed to the lower price and began dealing with the Colombians independently, using the operating capital which Suárez had given him to buy paste. Unable to sell his stock, Suárez was ruined.

Suárez struggled to salvage his empire, trying again to smuggle cocaine directly into the US. He sent the husband of his daughter Heidi, a man called Gerardo Caballero, to the US with 300 kilos of cocaine but Gerardo was caught and gaoled. Suárez responded by putting out a contract on the life of the US ambassador to Bolivia, Edwin Corr. Corr was swiftly pulled out and reassigned to a safer place: El Salvador.

Meanwhile, Suárez's grip on power was further undermined by a weakness for his own product. 'Suárez became one of his best customers,' says a DEA source.

Then came another bombshell. This time it came in the form of a video cassette which rapidly became known as the narco-video, or Bolivia's Watergate. In April 1988 a video was handed over to the Bolivian congress which showed a right-wing politician, a retired army general and a businessman at a *fiesta* with Suárez at his house in Santa Cruz. In the video, which had been filmed several years earlier, the guests drank and slapped each other on the shoulder as Robbie Suárez livened things up with some songs on the guitar. The only person aware he was being filmed was Suárez, who grinned at the camera.

What were the men doing with Suárez? Their excuses, delivered to Bolivia's congress in May 1988, made amusing listening.

Alfredo Arce Carpio, head of the parliamentary bench of the right-wing ADN party and interior minister under General Banzer, declared he had attended the meeting for 'journalistic reasons' but had been deeply disappointed. 'The man was a prisoner of his own ideas,' he said. 'He was a dethroned king who hoped to regain his kingdom.' No-one apparently saw fit to ask him how he had achieved such a rapid change of profession and why he had not published the results. Rafael Puente, leader of the Patriotic Alliance party, for one, was unconvinced. 'I don't think that a journalist, when he interviews somebody, hugs him with such overwhelming emotion.'

The retired army general, Mario Vargas Salinas, now a white-haired old man but formerly a prominent member of the forces fighting Che Guevara in the 1960s and minister of labour under Banzer, admitted he was a personal friend of 'The Godfather' but said he had visited Suárez to carry out a 'military investigation'. His aim was to check out for himself reports that Suárez's arsenal was bigger than that of the Bolivian army. Reporting on the 'results' of his 'investigation' to congress, he said he too had been disappointed. 'I didn't see his military advisers from Libya or the vertical take-off planes which Suárez had boasted about in press interviews,' he said. This version, however, failed to explain why, in the video, Vargas Salinas slaps Suárez on the shoulder saying 'Roberto, I admire you. You are a fine man.'

The third man, Jorge Alvéstegui, director of an advertising company, said he had attended the meeting to tie up some advertising business but refused to elaborate. 'After meeting Suárez, I concluded that the king of cocaine was a bluff,' he told congress.

No-one believed them. 'By their smiles, their friendship and their embraces, these three men showed that they were involved in drug trafficking and that a lot of ADN's finances came from these contacts,' declared union leader Filemón Escobar.

The La Paz rumour mill went wild. The most plausible explanation was that the meeting was arranged so that the three men could ask Suárez for money to buy off opposition members of parliament and senators to ensure the success of Banzer's ADN party in the 1985 elections. Suárez would probably have been well disposed towards the idea, since the government at the time, that of Siles Zuazo, had just taken harsh measures against his Beni cocaine labs and he was hungry for revenge. An inquiry later claimed to reveal that Suárez had offered $200,000 for the ADN's election campaign. Another version took the opposite view: that Suárez had filmed the meeting to humiliate the ADN and prevent their election victory because they had failed to give him promised protection. In other words, it was the desperate act of a man who knew he was no longer king. According to this version, Suárez knew Banzer had promised Washington that if he won the elections he would cooperate in fighting drugs.

Whatever the truth, no political party wanted to delve too deeply. For although the characters on the video were ADN members, Suárez hinted darkly that he had dozens more videos in his narcovideotheque which incriminated members of all parties. 'Uncle Robert', even if no longer king of cocaine, still had considerable power over politicians. If they took harsh measures against him, all he needed to do was pull out another video 'nasty'. To this day, fear of what secrets may be contained in Suárez's video library makes politicians hesitate to treat the cocaine chief too harshly.

Meanwhile, the Bolivian government was facing intense pressure from Washington to show it was serious about fighting drugs. Suárez was the obvious target. In early 1988, a judge sentenced Suárez to 15 years in gaol. He never showed up for his trial, so was tried, convicted and sentenced in his absence. Meanwhile, Bolivia's anti-drug police began scouring the Beni in one of the biggest drugs hunts in the country's history.

Other reports say Suárez was pursued as a result of pressure from Techo on instructions from Colombia's Medellín cartel who wanted to punish Suárez for his refusal to sell his cocaine at Colombian prices in 1984 and 1985. Techo allegedly saw his uncle's arrest as the best means of securing his position at the head of a drugs empire which stretched to Mexico, Brazil, the US and Europe.

At 10.00 p.m. on Monday 18 July 1988, a 12-man police patrol arrived on foot at Suárez's Quemalia ranch. Only two members of the patrol knew who they were looking for. Walking by night and hiding by day, they crept across the dusty plains of the Beni. The police could not use helicopters because their noise would give the game away.

At six o'clock two days later they reached another ranch called El Sujo, 35 kilometres from the town of Trinidad. They surrounded the house.

'By luck Suárez was in there,' says one of the anti-drugs police who took part in the raid.

> It was a friend's birthday so Suárez had not been quite as careful about security as he'd normally be. Usually, before he goes to a house he sends his bodyguards to spy it out and only goes if he gets the all-clear. He has about 20 bodyguards, all armed with high-calibre rifles. There are Lebanese ex-terrorists, Brazilians, Colombians. As we arrived at the house, Suárez was resting. When the security guards saw us they radioed 'The Leopards are here.' A short shootout followed, but nobody was hurt. All but two of the bodyguards ran for it, abandoning Suárez with his wife and sons.

The police captured 25 sophisticated firearms and a number of videos and photographs, but not a trace of dope.

The police flew Suárez to Trinidad, the capital of the Beni, but decided that security in the gaol was inadequate for a trafficker of Suárez's standing. The Americans wanted Suárez extradited to the US but the government refused. Instead Suárez was flown the next day to La Paz and taken to the headquarters of the anti-narcotics police.

Suárez, used to the steamy heat of the low-lying Beni, found it difficult to adapt to the 12,000-foot altitude of the Bolivian capital. He had to be given emergency medical treatment for a heart condition and the police lent him a parka to keep him warm. Suárez asked to be allowed to stay at headquarters because, he said, at the prison there could be reprisals from other traffickers. The request was turned down.

Six days after his arrest, Suárez climbed calmly out of the red police car which had stopped outside the green iron gates of San Pedro prison. The *plaza* in front was packed with residents, journalists and passers-by who had been waiting since dawn to witness the legend. As Suárez passed they threw him food and cheered as if he had been the president. As the gaol door slammed shut, a cry went up from the prisoners inside: 'Long Live the King.'

A few days later, journalists packed into a room near Suárez's cell.

'I agreed to this press conference on the understanding that you will not distort it, for the theme we are talking about [drug trafficking] is delicate and extremely risky,' declared Suárez, shaking with nerves and wearing six days of stubble. Risky for whom? wondered the journalists. 'Before we start I want to ask you if you really realise the criminality involved in drug trafficking. I want one of you to talk about the subject to ensure we treat it with respect and responsibility.' A journalist retorted that they had come to hear Suárez not themselves. The druglord apologised.

> I am not a pedant or a cretin.... With all due modesty I can say I am the only person on this earth capable of fighting drug trafficking. ['Why? Mr Suárez,' asked one journalist.] Because I went to school. ['The school of drug trafficking?'] That's it. You need to go to school if you want to learn and I went to ' school to learn, OK? What I'd like to do is to make a loud call to Reagan and his government; it's not a pardon plea because I don't fall on my knees before any man, but I do so before the Creator who is the only one who has the power to forgive or punish. It is possible that I, given the respect that the President of Bolivia owes me, might ask him a special favour: that the north American government together with judicial representatives present its case against me, here, in my country.

Moving from the quirky to the ridiculous, Suárez said he wanted a trial by Grand Jury, attended by the pope. The journalists scribbled down the quotes in their notebooks.

Meanwhile, police investigating Suárez's case went to the bank vaults in La Paz, where the ledgers and records confiscated from Suárez's ranch, which showed details of cocaine deals and flights, had been put. They had disappeared.

So ended the biggest anti-drugs operation in Bolivia's history. Or was it?

Suárez himself has another version: that he gave himself up and went to gaol to prove his innocence. 'I knew exactly what time the police had set out and what time they were arriving,' he told journalists. 'I was dressed and smoking a cigarette when they arrived. I had decided to let them capture me.... I facilitated my capture precisely because I could not continue to carry the guilt of traffickers on my shoulders.'

Suárez's capture was almost certainly the result of a deal. For years, the authorities had known where the kingpin was but failed to arrest him for fear he might compromise certain members of the government. US pressure finally forced their hand. What the government gave Suárez to ensure his silence will never be known. Some reports say it was simply a promise not to extradite him or an agreement to let him off after a few years. Others say huge sums were paid.

SUAREZ, used to the huge open spaces of the Beni, felt like a caged lion in his cold cramped prison cell. He missed his horses, the fuchsia sunsets, the smell of freshly barbecued steak. The only things that made life bearable were the daily newspapers and presents sent to him by Robbie, one of the few members of his family who remembered him. Sometimes he even got in the odd bottle of whisky. According to one prisoner, Robbie also helped his father plot a military coup to avenge his imprisonment. One evening in 1989, Suárez was watching a comedy on television. It was suddenly interrupted with the news that Robbie had been shot.

It turned out to have been an accident. One evening three or four police officers had arrived at the Santa Cruz house of Robbie's stunning girl friend, Carmiña Ortiz, the former wife of the racing car driver, Carlos Hugo 'Chino' Mendez, who had been killed in a crash. They rang the doorbell and a child let them in. Inside they found Robbie slouched on a chair and Carmiña and her sister Ruth in hammocks. It is unclear who fired first.

According to Suárez senior, Carmiña tried to repel the police but was brushed aside by Robbie who said he would 'speak with the *señores*'. The police then shot him in the neck and stomach. A version given by one of the policemen who was wounded is that the police tried to arrest Robbie but that he tried to shoot. In the commotion he fell and Ruth picked up the pistol and shot at the policeman saying, 'We have to kill these bastards'. The policeman was wounded on his left shoulder.

News of his son's death came as a bitter blow to Suárez, who became afraid he would be kidnapped by druglords to whom he owed debts. Prison security was stepped up drastically.

Today, Suárez muses how long he will wait before spilling the beans. 'I'm giving them until the end of the year [1991] to give me justice, then I'll talk. People in the Bolivian government and the US embassy tremble when they come to see me. They are terrified what I might say.' In reality he knows he is safer inside than out. And according to some reports he no longer has the wealth to pay his way out. One prisoner claims Suárez owes hundreds of dollars for food alone and is frantically trying to sell his *narco*-videos.

Most prisoners can pay their way out with a bribe of around $2,000. But Suárez is too big; it would be impossible for his escape to go unnoticed, and the costs for the Bolivian government in terms of international credibility would be huge.

'The most likely is that once he's got some cash, Suárez will give a judge $1 million or so in return for declaring his case a case of mistaken identity,' says a prison inmate. 'Then he'll walk out like a respectable *señor*. Alternatively, the government may declare his heart condition got worse and that he's dead.'

A knock is heard at the door. A guard enters timidly and says there is a visitor for Don Roberto. A thin man with a Hitler-style moustache comes into the room, eyes up the unexpected visitors and whispers something to Suárez. He excuses himself and the two walk outside into the courtyard for a private chat. 'He's from the interior ministry,' explains Suárez's wife who reluctantly leaves her sewing machine to keep me busy. 'You know Suárez doesn't like journalists very much: they always distort things. He hasn't let one in here for over a year.'

She sighs, and turns her hostile eyes towards me. 'I don't know how much longer I can stand it being stuck in here. I feel as if I'll explode one of these days.' Motioning to the figures on the bed, she adds: 'Can you imagine bringing up two kids in a single room, never seeing the daylight? It's no life for them.'

Suárez returns alone and takes another bottle of Pepsi out of the fridge. 'You tell the British government they're doing a great job. It's vital they control the drugs trade and don't let impure drugs fall into the hands of delinquents.'

He lapses into philosophical mood. 'I don't hate anybody. What bothers me is the lack of justice. Even Bush. You may be surprised but I don't even hate him. When I get out of here, I just want to go back to my cattle. I've always been a rancher and that's all I want to do. I've thought about politics, but I've had enough.'

The interview is over and Suárez ushers me to the prison gate. He stares wistfully at the bustling street outside. 'Give Margaret a kiss from me.'

4

Turning a Blind Eye:
The Police

Chimoré

CAPTAIN Jorge Saavedra stops his battered red Toyota truck beside a cluster of corrugated-iron huts in the village of Paractito, a few kilometres up a dirt track off the main Cochabamba to Santa Cruz road. His eight uniformed men tumble out of the back, slinging their M-16 submachine guns over their shoulders. A few villagers stare sullenly at the intruders while chickens peck around their feet. They pretend to look uninterested, but undisguised hatred is written in their eyes.

Jorge pulls a screwed up scrap of yellow paper out of the pocket of his uniform and spreads it out on the bonnet of the truck. On it is scrawled a primitive map, like a child's drawing of a treasure hunt.

'At the houses we need to take the path to the river where there should be a suspension bridge,' he says, mopping the early morning sweat from his forehead. 'Then we turn left along the main track beside the river. After a few hundred yards we branch left down a smaller path. The first pit should be there.'

The men, nicknamed the Leopards because of their spotted fatigues, belong to Bolivia's élite anti-narcotics police officially known as UMOPAR (*Unidad Móbil de Patrullaje Rural* or Mobile Rural Patrol Unit). They are based at Chimoré, one hour's drive away.

The map was drawn by an informant who stole into the barracks in the night. Depending on whether the Leopards find any paste or base, the man, who works at one of the targeted pits, may earn anything from $10 to $100. Sometimes informants come out on raids with the Leopards. They dress up in camouflage uniform, make up their faces and carry machine guns, although unlike those of the Leopards they are not loaded. If discovered by their masters, though, the price is instant death at the hands of special death squads. Today's informant has decided not to risk it.

A gunshot echoes through the dense jungle canopy on the other side of the river: the traffickers obviously got wind of the raid long before the Leopards arrived and are warning people to leg it. Walkie-talkie operators along the main road almost certainly alerted them when they saw the UMOPAR truck leaving Chimoré, or police at checkpoints *en route* tipped them off. On hearing the signal, workers at the maceration pits flee to the village with the paste and play football until the police have left.

Jorge turns to the driver who is staying behind to guard the truck. 'We'll be gone a couple of hours,' he says. 'I don't think the traffickers are armed, but if you hear three shots, come and find us.' Looking at Jorge you cannot tell he is a captain, for he is dressed exactly like everyone else. 'You don't display your rank,' he explains. 'If you did the *narcos* would make a bee-line for you.'

Crossing the river is not as easy as the map implies. As often happens the informant forgot to mention a crucial detail: the absence of a bridge. Following heavy rains the night before, the river has turned into an angry torrent and the only means of crossing is a rusty iron rope which once supported a suspension bridge. The Leopards plunge in up to their waists and clumsily haul themselves to the far bank. Unperturbed at being sodden to their underpants, they forge into the jungle like a trail of tropical green ants.

Turning left along a wide jungle track, they reach a bamboo house on stilts. The Leopard in front kicks the door open and searches it. There is nobody inside. A few yards further, however, they spot the first tell-tale signs: a bed made out of bamboo sticks, protected by white polythene sheeting suspended from the trees above. Makeshift beds like this are used by workers at the pits.

As the police reach another house, a young man with dark curly hair strolls out. He is barefoot and wears a filthy pair of navy trousers with no flies and a T-shirt which says 'I love New York'. Realising he is trapped, he stares sullenly at the mud floor.

'You're doped, aren't you?' Jorge asks.

'No,' mutters the youth.

'What have you been doing?'

'Just harvesting coca leaves.'

'Liar,' Jorge replies, handcuffing the man's hands behind his back with a plastic cord. 'I'm going to tighten the handcuffs. Talk and I'll let you go.'

'How can I talk if I don't know anything?' protests the youth. 'What are you going to do to me?'

'I know you're working in drugs. If you talk later it'll be too late. Do you want to collaborate?'

'But I don't know anything.'

'Your feet are dirty. You were stomping coca last night.'

'No, that's just water. There's a river further along the path.'

Another Leopard uses his machine gun to prod a cooking pot whose sloppy brown contents are still warm. Strewn on the dirt floor beside it is a pile of muddy cassava roots, a bowl of peeled onions and carrots, and a bag of toilet rolls.

'You've been cooking, it seems,' says Jorge. 'Who owns the house?' Often traffickers rent houses from local people so they can be tracked down less easily, and move on to another spot a few days later, according to the intensity of police raids.

'He's called Alberto.'

'Liar. What's your name?'

'Estéfano Botosí.'

Two other policeman who went off to search the area join the group with another bedraggled youth in handcuffs, presumably another stomper.

'Take us to the pits,' they order the men, prodding them in the back with their M-16s. Jorge chips in. 'By the way, if you should think of escaping, there are three more Leopard patrols near here.'

Perched between the river and the jungle, the pit, or *pozo*, consists of a basin of white plastic sheeting containing a lethal tea-coloured brew of coca leaves, water and kerosene. At the far end are two small separate compartments, or *chicleros*, where the extracted *agua rica* (rich water) is mixed with more, even more lethal, chemicals. A stinking mass of brown coca leaves is heaped along the far edge. On the near side are big blue and orange plastic tubs containing the paste's vital chemical ingredients, a saucepan of still-warm lentil soup, and some small plastic bags of coca leaves, chewed by the stompers to keep themselves going.

Jorge turns to his companions who are kicking the plastic drums in search of drugs. 'The drugs have gone,' he says. 'The people probably took them with them when they fled, or buried them in secret hiding places in the jungle. There were six people working here, including my informant.'

He summons the two youths. 'Show us how you stomp the leaves or you'll remember it tonight.'

Still handcuffed, the boys step sulkily into the fetid mixture and walk spiritlessly up and down, pounding the leaves with their ulcerated bare feet. It is a sad contrast to how it must have been a few hours earlier, dancing frenziedly, and secure in the cover of the night.

The task accomplished, the policemen cut the boys' plastic handcuffs with their machetes. Estéfano squirms with pain as one policeman pierces his wrist instead.

The Leopards prepare a great bonfire. Everything, from the chemicals to the white sheet roof to the little bags of coca leaves, is hurled onto the huge pile. Only the largest plastic containers are retrieved: they will be useful in the Chimoré kitchens as washing-up bowls or as presents to charity organisations.

But there is one thing the Leopards did not foresee. When the time comes to ignite the pyre, they discover the river crossing has turned their box of US-made matches into a soggy cardboard ball. The captain dips a pair of underpants he has found into the kerosene mixture, hoists it on the end of a bamboo pole and shoots at it with his M-16. The surrounding trees shudder but not a spark emerges. He fires twice more in vain.

'Go and find some matches,' he orders.

The Leopards climb a steep trail and emerge again onto the main track. A short way along they find another one-roomed hut. The door is open and its contents strewn over the floor as if its inhabitants left in a hurry. Inside, it stinks of urine. On one side is a bamboo bed, piled with sordid children's clothes and a pillow. On the floor are a saucepan of peeled potatoes and more tell-tale packets of toilet paper. A Leopard finally finds a packet of matches and a cigarette lighter on the ledge by the door. He grabs them and the toilet rolls. 'These rolls will come in useful at the barracks,' he mutters, suspending them from his US-army belt.

The midday heat is beginning to get intense and the men are anxious to get on with the job. Returning to the pit they order the two prisoners to pour on the last barrel of kerosene. They set light to the kerosene-soaked rag and throw it onto the bonfire. With a huge explosion, hundreds of dollars worth of chemicals and equipment are consumed in a mass of flame. For the Leopards, it is part of an ordinary day's work. For the traffickers, a minor loss to set against their profits.

On the way back to the truck the Leopards stop off at the stompers' house to let them pick up a spare pair of trousers and a blanket. Just before returning to the river they meet an old man and a barefooted Indian woman wearing a brightly coloured shawl. The man's left cheek bulges with coca leaves.

'Have you got an identity card?' Jorge asks him.

'No,' says the man nervously.

'What about her?'

'She doesn't speak Spanish.'

From her bewildered looks, it is clear the woman is a Quechua or Aymara Indian. The captain dismisses the pair with his hand.

'You can go,' he says.

'Thank you very much, sir,' says the man, hurrying away before the captain can change his mind. Jorge turns to his companions. 'If these people are unbothered, it's because they're not in drugs. Those folks have all gone to the mountain. These people know where they are, but they don't talk. If they talk, they'd be killed.'

Back at Paractito, the stompers are loaded like cattle into the floor of the back of the truck, surveyed by the Leopards who perch on the seats. Realising what is to come, one of them, Estéfano, begins to plead pathetically with the captain.

'Please let me go. I'm just a poor *campesino*. Don't take me to prison.'

'Don't worry. We'll see the *fiscal* [public prosecutor] when we get to Chimoré and maybe he'll let you off,' replies the captain, climbing into the front of the truck. As a simple stomper the youth knows he will probably get one or two years in prison. His bosses meanwhile will be wandering around town untouched, respectable *señores*.

At the base camp in Chimoré, it is nearly time for lunch and the other Leopards are either relaxing in the main exercise yard after a morning sortie or playing basketball on the pitch behind the sleeping quarters. From time to time trucks roar in and unload their cargo of UMOPAR agents and coca paste wrapped in black plastic bags. The drugs are stored in a special store-room to which only the top two officers have the key.

As Captain Saavedra's truck draws in, two policeman posted outside the prison cells reluctantly interrupt a game of dice to deal with the captives. They line them up against the wall with their hands behind their heads, and frisk them. The cell doors are then unlocked and the boys shoved inside a dark room where three ghost-like figures are peeling potatoes into a huge iron cauldron. The youths slump onto a couple of mattresses, a mixture of indifference and despair on their faces. The policemen yawn, lock the gates and return to their game. There is one thing both policeman and prisoner understands: had the captives been Big Fish, they would not be there.

THE FIRST sign that you have reached Chimoré base camp is a checkpoint on the main Cochabamba-Santa Cruz highway where unsmiling UMOPAR agents wave down passing vehicles and check them for dope or precursors. Sometimes the search is thorough: they even check the inside of the engine and the tyres. Sometimes they ask for money instead.

Behind the checkpoint, an electronic barrier leads to the camp's white-washed prefabricated huts which are dotted across a wide jungle clearing. Near the entrance is the trophy of a recent raid: the charred wing of a Cessna plane, abandoned and burned by traffickers as they saw the police approach. At the far end, two droning helicopters lift off from the airstrip and drift away over the jungle canopy like two huge black flying beetles.

Life in Chimoré, as in any South American army or police camp, is a combination of regimented tedium, *machismo* and round-the-clock activity. Up at 6.00, the Leopards spend their day patrolling areas like the Red Zone, or raiding secret paste pits or labs following tip-offs from informants. If it is a big raid, US DEA agents come too, officially to advise, but effectively to run the operation.

Around 380 of UMOPAR's total 640 personnel are based here, the rest being posted in the Beni. They are recruited from the Bolivian national police and come under the control of the La Paz-based Special Force for the

Fight Against Drug Trafficking. They are supplemented by a 150-man air wing recruited from the Bolivian Air Force, known as the Red Devils, and by a 75-member force from the Bolivian Navy which works mainly on the rivers of the Beni.

On the right-hand side of the base, behind their own wire fence, are the living quarters of the camp's other residents, the DEA and US Special Forces. All are participants in the principal US anti-cocaine effort in the Andes, Operation Snowcap.

'Welcome to the Chapare Safari', reads a notice over the door of the hut which serves as the day room for the 20 or so DEA agents. Inside fair-haired agents in khaki T-shirts and trousers drink imported 7-Up and plan the next raid as the local cook prepares the evening's supper; today as a change from mince, she is making meat loaf, a recipe taught to her by the DEA's only female agent here, Roz. On the sofa in front of the television the cook's seven-year-old son is slumped asleep. On the wall is a For Sale notice. 'Hookworms. Nice Pets', it reads. 'Easy to care for. Eat what you eat. Go where you go. Interested? Contact Dave Mitchell.'

Next door are the dormitories. Photographs of girlfriends and nude pin-ups plaster the walls behind the neat rows of mosquito net-covered bunks. Under the beds the agents store their medals, love letters and food hampers from Mom. A few blocks along is the weights room, nicknamed the *Casa del Dolor* (House of Pain). Its little back room houses the DEA pets: a python called Natasha, a parrot called Harry, and a hen. 'Her name is dinner,' says an agent.

The accommodation is a great improvement on what the DEA had before: 'In 1987 we just had tents and wooden shacks and only had baths every five days,' remembers Tom, a DEA medic. 'We drank out of the well and ate in the *comedor* with the Leopards. The food was disgusting: there were literally worms in the sauce. I'd have to eat a MRE [Meal Ready to Eat] afterwards. We used to say we were wearing "green socks"; that meant we always had diarrhoea. What we have now is Club Med in comparison.'

A more discreet presence is kept by US Special Forces personnel who live opposite in separate quarters, and who even have a different cook. Special Forces personnel, whose exact number is kept a secret but is around 15, tend to be older and more taciturn than the DEA temporary agents and have little contact with them except on Sundays when they take it in turns to prepare a joint barbecue. They live by stricter rules too, including a ban on alcohol except for a bottle of beer on Friday and Saturday nights. In La Paz, military personnel are even forbidden to drink coca tea, regardless of the fact that it is far less harmful than tobacco or alcohol.

In Chimoré they provide logistical and planning back-up to the DEA and give small-unit tactical training to UMOPAR at the base's training school, the Escuela de Garras del Valor (Brave Claws School). The school, set up with US aid in May 1987, initially provided training to officers but now extends to all ranks as well as to police from neighbouring countries. Selected UMOPAR personnel are also sent for training at Fort Benning, Georgia, in the US.

Special Forces medics also run a clinic on the base which is one of the best in the Chapare. The clinic is part of US efforts to 'pacify' the area and convince local people that repression is not their only aim. Until recently it treated as many as 40 people a day, many of whom came from as far away as Cochabamba. Most suffer from tuberculosis, or respiratory and intestinal problems. The clinic's chief medic, Randy Richie, points to a row of bottles displaying some of the more gruesome objects which have been found inside his patients' bodies. There's a round worm several metres long, a family of maggots and even a wodge of coca leaves which were found stuffed inside one old man's ear to cure his earache. 'We've delivered 11 babies here, too,' he says. Now fewer locals come here, partly because the Bolivian police are setting up clinics themselves in local towns, but also according to one account because US tax-payers could not see the point.

The clinic does serve one important law enforcement purpose though: it acts as a cover-up for informants. The medics give them prescriptions and a bottle of vitamin pills to take away with them. Sometimes they stay overnight in one of the clinic's tiny closets for questioning.

COLONEL Rogelio Vargas, the *comandante,* tastes a spoonful of a stew, a watery *mélange* of gristly meat, over-cooked carrots and gelatinous white rice, and tops it with a dollop of tomato ketchup. UMOPAR food, prepared by the camp's cook with the help of female prisoners, is brought to him in the officers' mess every mealtime for him to test. He nods to the trooper hovering at his side. 'It's OK,' he says, probably thinking otherwise.

Vargas, a soft-spoken man with velvet brown eyes and a baby face, has tasted a few UMOPAR dinners in his time. A policeman for nearly 30 years, he has taken part in some of the country's most dramatic raids, from the capture in 1989 of Arce Gómez, the so-called 'Minister of Cocaine', to Operation Blast Furnace in 1986 when 180 US military joined UMOPAR forces in a major blitz against the traffickers.

He nods mechanically as a group of officers who have just entered wish him an optimistic *buen provecho* (have a good meal) and serve themselves from big iron cauldrons. Outside the mosquito-netting windows, the song of crickets can just be heard above the clatter from the troop's mess next door. Lowering his voice to a soft murmur, he tells his story:

> When I first arrived in the Chapare, I went to the Red Zone to look around. One day at around 4.00 in the afternoon, I went into Isinuta which at that time was totally controlled by the traffickers. I disguised my face and wore a hat and a pair of old jeans so they'd think I was just a local lad. I hadn't washed for several days

before, so they wouldn't think I was suspiciously clean. And I had to go unarmed because if they found weapons they would know immediately I was a cop. As I went into the village, a man asked me, 'What are you doing?' I said I was looking for a friend who was 'working', that's the slang for 'he's in drugs'. I used a Santa Cruz accent which I'd been practising for weeks before. I knew if I didn't get it right I'd die. Then the man asked me my name. I knew no-one ever had names. If I'd said 'I'm looking for Pedro X,' they'd have smelt a rat immediately. So I said I was looking for *El Negro* [The Dark One]. I did my recce without problems and got out unscathed.

The traffickers keep meticulously close tabs on us with their walkie-talkies. They follow us everywhere. They know every detail of my personal life, even the colour of my cars. Sometimes I take a different car to fool them, but they soon catch on. You have no privacy. Wherever I go, people say 'There goes the *comandante*.' If I go to a bar or a restaurant I have to be very careful who I mix with. If I chat up a young woman, for example, people assume I am telling her secrets about the traffickers or that she's an informant. That could cause her serious problems. The traffickers also use attractive girls to seduce me and get me to take bribes, so I have to be wary when I meet nice women. I have to be cold and firm.

The traffickers buy their walkie-talkies in Santa Cruz or Cochabamba. They're good quality, particularly the Japanese ones. I've captured a couple, so I listen to them to see what they're up to. They speak at the same time every day, always using code. They give us all names. Places have nicknames too. I'm Number One. When we are going into the Red Zone, they say 'He's going towards the castle.' When we hear nothing we know they've not seen us coming. Or they say 'All white'. That means 'All clear'. Nothing's ever called by its real name. A machine gun, for example, is 'toaster'. For dope they have hundreds of names: *pilcha* [garment], *pichicata*, *merca* [merchandise], *cola de pez* [fish tail] or 'orange'. Because of our green uniforms, they call us 'parrots' or 'banana growers', or 'fishermen'. Our trucks are 'canoes'. If a black one passes, they say, 'There goes the widow.' The choppers they call 'hair cutters' or '*tocotocos*', from the sound they make. Infiltration is 'egg'; when they realise they've been infiltrated, they say 'the chicken has laid some eggs'. Among themselves, too, the traffickers avoid using real names so that they can't be identified. Instead they use nicknames like *Techo de Paja* [Thatch Roof], *Caballo Loco* [Crazy Horse] or *El Gallo* [The Rooster].

The traffickers used to avoid working at night because they were afraid of assaults and murders. Now they have to because we don't let them work by day. It makes it difficult for their planes to take off. Sometimes the drugs go bad. Recently they've started using special coloured reflectors to help them see the drugs. If we went in at night, we could get them, but it's too dangerous: they shoot at anything. We only go to a place at night if we've got information and we're sure there's something there. It's ironic: I used to be very afraid of the dark. When I was a child I would hang onto my mother when night fell. Now I'm used to it. In any case, I have to accompany my troops.

Almost all our operations are based on tip-offs from informants. They come into the barracks at night, so no-one will see them, and knock on my bedroom window. We put balaclavas on their heads and cover up any tattoos on their arms so no-one in the base will recognise them. If they're too scared to come here, they send a child or wife to arrange a secret meeting place in the jungle. Often the informant is a worker at a lab. He sneaks out to meet me somewhere on the road at an agreed time and tells me about the lab, then slips back to his folks a few hours later. Nobody suspects where he's been. I wait until I get two reports about a particular lab before acting on it; that way you can check them against each other and make sure they're not lying. The amount we pay them depends on what we find. If, for example, we find ten kilos of paste, he might get $200. If the tip-off leads to the arrest of a major trafficker, he could get $5,000. On average, an informant earns around $20 for every kilo found. Sometimes we have problems because we run out of money and we can't pay them. It's not our fault, it's that the government hasn't sent it through. If the information is good, we'll use the guy again. We have a list of the reliable ones.

It's risky for them of course. If a guy is found out he will certainly be killed. Only last week in Voltadero, an hour's drive north of here, an informant was beaten to death then hacked into pieces as a warning. The assassins left a note on his body saying 'This is how informants die.' We had 21 guys in here accused of taking part in the killing. Sometimes informants have to move out of the area to save their lives.

The way to catch the *narcos* is to infiltrate them. We've got a number of ways. Sometimes we go out in an ordinary-looking lorry with a double floor. Into the top we load sacks of coca leaves, some food and some lime, so they think we're going to make drugs. We put our cook with the sacks, disguised as an Indian woman, and tell her to chew coca so she looks convincing. We use a prisoner as a driver: if he agrees to take part in the game, we let him off. Meanwhile, my men are crouched in the bottom of the lorry, ready to leap out when they hear the signal.

Last week we used this method for a night raid on Isinuta where we knew there was a stash of 1,200 kilos of coca paste, divided into three loads of 700, 400 and 100 kilos. This time, though, the decoy was the UMOPAR themselves: we had three lorries. Each had six visible men up top, plus another four hidden below. We took the road to San Francisco, about two hours' drive from here. As we left Chimoré, I listened to my radio and waited for the traffickers to count us out. The voice came: 'There are three canoes going out. Six in each. All white.' They hadn't realised that in fact there were ten in each lorry. About half an hour before San Francisco, one of the Leopards gave the colour torch signal which meant the infiltrators were to leap out in 60 seconds. One man in each lorry had been assigned to watch for the signal.

When it was time, the infiltrators, including me, silently leapt out and hid in the undergrowth beside the track. I listened nervously to my radio: 'All white, they're going on to San Francisco.' I heaved a sigh of relief as I saw the lorries speeding on to San Francisco to carry out what the traffickers thought was a routine patrol.

By now it was about 2.00 a.m. and it had started to rain. I was armed and had food and water, but was terribly cold. We crept up a very small path in the direction of Isinuta, careful to avoid snakes. We could hardly see anything but it was too dangerous to light a torch: the *narcos* would have instantly seen us and fired. Unfortunately we don't have any night vision equipment, so we use cats eyes you know, the things they put on roads to help drivers at night, which each man has on the back of his cap. From two until dawn we hacked through thick jungle to the Isinuta road. By now, I was soaked through and tired and all I could think of was bed.

Suddenly a dog barked just 50 metres away. The enemy was right next to us, only separated by a barbed wire fence. We froze, praying the dogs would shut up. Nobody fired. I suppose they were too surprised, just couldn't imagine it could be us. The rain pattered on. The next thing was to make a radio link with my informant who we had arranged would be buying drugs from the traffickers at this time. But the informant had decided it would be too risky to be seen carrying his walkie-talkie. So he did a very clever thing. Earlier he had drunk something to make him as sick as a dog, and had hidden his walkie-talkie up the road inside some trees. As soon as the traffickers started buying drugs, the man rushed off holding his stomach and throwing up and went to where the walkie-talkie was hidden. He grabbed it and messaged me. 'They're buying,' he said. 'Hold your guns,' I replied. My main object was the 700-kilo stash. I knew exactly which house it was in, but it wasn't going to be easy. The streets are narrow and almost impossible to enter without being seen. The *narcos* were monitoring every movement on the road from Chimoré, but luckily it hadn't occurred to them to take care of the jungle on the right of the village where we were. My next problem was to make sure the helicopters left Chimoré at exactly the right time. The traffickers would be able to hear them half an hour before they got to Isinuta so it was vital they didn't set out too early or the whole thing would be ruined. I listened to my radio to check when the choppers were leaving.

Suddenly the radio went dead. The rain had cut off the contact. I now had to rely on our back-up plan which was that if the helicopters got no message they would arrive at noon. It was now 11.25. We had five minutes in which to act. We rushed into the village. Three shots went off — someone was selling drugs. I entered the house where the 400-kilo stash was and seized a black plastic bag of paste. Then an extraordinary thing happened: a fire broke out in that very building. Being policemen as well as anti-drug agents we were obliged by law to put the fire out. Meanwhile, the *narcos* all fled with their drugs. A few minutes earlier we'd have got them red-handed.

We policemen have a saying: 'The *narcos* have a *narco* god who always helps them.' The traffickers seem to have an inordinate share of good luck. We, on the other hand, seem to have an inordinate share of bad. Perhaps it's because the *narcos* take care to appease the spirits. They are extremely superstitious. They kill birds and wear amulets to protect themselves and to make sure business goes well. Some of them wash in special aromatic potions to bring themselves luck. Others scatter beer on the ground or carry mascot dolls. They're also very devout Catholics, though of course they only practise when it suits them.

One of our biggest hauls was in 1987 in the department of Santa Cruz. We were flying over the jungle and saw an airstrip with a big stash on it. There were several boxes with a plank on top and a woman was looking after them. We landed and asked her what she was doing there. 'I don't know what's in these boxes, *comandante*,' she said. 'I was just told to guard them till the plane comes to collect them.' We examined the boxes, but then realised the traffickers would smell a rat if they had been moved. The trouble was, we couldn't remember what position they'd been in originally. Suddenly we heard the plane approaching. The most important thing was to occupy the woman's hands so she wouldn't give a signal to the trafficker. I told her to clutch the boxes so they wouldn't notice they'd been moved.

We had hardly had time to run for cover when the plane landed. When the trafficker touched the ground and saw us he accelerated and tried to take off again straight away. I thought he was going to squash us like mosquitoes. Luckily I managed to shoot him in the leg. 'Don't kill me,' he yelled as he fell. I questioned him. He was carrying the drugs from Puerto Aurora in the Chapare to a *hacienda* in Santa Cruz. We picked him up and flew him to a clinic. He was hysterical and was sure we were going to throw him out of the plane. He was later sentenced to six years, although he should have got 20, but unfortunately he got out a few days later.

The DEA considers Colonel Vargas one of the cleanest police officers in Bolivia. But the distinction, while it earns Vargas brownie points and essential aid from the US, can bring bitter retribution from traffickers and from colleagues and government officials who protect them. They fear Vargas, by refusing bribes, will show them up. Other clean police officers complain they are shunned by peers and deliberately passed over for promotion. 'If you act honestly, you are seen as a nuisance,' says one officer, who asked not to be named. 'They say "He's not one of us. He's harming us."' Some have had their lives, and those of their families, threatened. Vargas, who has one of the choicest posts in Bolivia in terms of kickbacks, is almost certain that, were it not for US pressure, he would have been transferred long ago.

Vargas is the exception to the rule. The profits to be made in cocaine are so huge that few policemen can resist the bribes offered them unless they have private means. High-ranking ones have regular protection payments put into their bank accounts, or receive handsome one-off sums in return for allowing a plane to land. One commander says he is offered $10,000 every four days to look the other way. Others actively participate in the cocaine industry, carrying chemicals or paste, distributing cocaine or supervising labs. Low-ranking police use raids to seize drugs which they resell, or to ransack *campesino* homes for money and valuables. Only when a trafficker can offer nothing is he arrested and used as evidence that drug raids are being taken seriously. 'Cocaine trafficking has prostituted our forces,' admitted General Elías Gutiérrez, commander of the Special Force Against Drug Trafficking, in mid-1991. '[The traffickers] have penetrated our forces at every level.'

For most a posting in the Chapare is a once in a lifetime chance to escape the trap of poverty and make a lot of money as fast as possible. A trooper earns a derisory 60 bucks a month, a top-ranking officer a maximum of 90. In addition, the US embassy gives monthly supplements of around $40 as an insurance against bribes. According to some US reports, however, many police have their base pay cut after being assigned to the Chapare, leaving them dependent on the supplement and whatever they can earn from bribes or stealing.

Corruption usually begins at the top. The commander may have been installed by a corrupt government official to whom he will pay a percentage cut of his kickbacks. Another portion may be distributed among the commander's subordinates. 'A commander might share out about 20 per cent of his extra earnings and keep 80 per cent for himself,' says a high-ranking police source. The commander and his colleagues ensure that corruption permeates the system below so that no-one will have cause to show them up. Corruption is installed in the trooper from the day he enters the force, says the source.

> The man at the top gives the man below him some 'help'. The young man knows if he doesn't accept he will be thrown out. And what will he do living on the street? So he takes it and says nothing. He doesn't ask where the money comes from. Already he's victim of a corrupt system in which you can't say No.

For a trooper like 30-year-old Roberto, working in the Chapare may be the only opportunity he will ever have to make life a little better for his wife and two children, five and four years old. Watched by his superior at a distance, he described his experience:

> I'm originally from Cochabamba but my family lives in La Paz. Unfortunately, being stuck here I rarely get a chance to see them. Apart from being far away, it's expensive to get to La Paz. I have to give all my earnings to the family. My children's schooling costs 60 *bolivianos* a month [$17] and the rent for the house in La Paz is 120 [$35]. I only earn 200 *bolivianos* [$60], so you see it doesn't leave much over. I can't afford to buy extra food (the food they give you here is fit only for animals) or clothes. If I wash my uniform, for example, I have to wear my underpants while it's drying. When I get my wages, I send them straight to the wife without even opening the pay packet. I can't even spend two *bolivianos* [55 US cents] on a Coca Cola.
>
> So you see it's a hard life being a UMOPAR policeman. I do it because I like my uniform, and at least it's some sort of a career. But if there was anything else I'd do it. We all would. So how do I survive? Well, you've guessed, corruption. There's lots of it. But if I tell you too much they'll take me by the ear to La Paz and my career will be kaput. But it's very difficult for them to control corruption here when we're all in the same boat. Imagine what you would do. If we go out on a raid and a trafficker shows us a $100 bill, with the few resources we have, what do you think we do? We think of our families. We take the money.... I have to stop talking, the colonel is coming.

Much of the corruption occurs at road checkpoints where police theoretically check passing vehicles for drugs, chemicals and contraband. In reality, they are bribe payment points. The amounts vary according to the rank of the police official and the passer-by. A low-level official, for instance, might charge a mere $10 to allow a small-time trafficker to take through a bundle of illegal coca leaves or precursors. His superior, on the other hand, might expect several thousand dollars for a large shipment of cocaine, particularly if the trafficker is a big fish. Sometimes police manning checkpoints fire on fellow Leopards and DEA agents to stop them carrying out anti-drug patrols. The DEA agents say they often have to run through checkpoints to prevent police having time to telephone traffickers to tip them off. No-one has yet been killed, but one DEA agent says he believes it is only a matter of time.

In September 1989, corruption at one checkpoint on the main Cochabamba-Santa Cruz road got so bad that the US embassy suspended salary supplements to a 30-man UMOPAR detachment for two months. Since the late 1980s, the US has been sending border patrol agents to help man checkpoints and search vehicles. But the agents acknowledge that their work is largely futile because the traffickers simply by-pass the checkpoints by walking through the jungle. The only checkpoints considered operational are those at either end of the valley. Bolivian police at checkpoints acknowledge they only clean up their act when US agents are around. When the Americans move elsewhere, or go on leave, things go back to normal. In March 1989, for example, a team of US border patrol agents assigned to a checkpoint at the entrance to the Chapare valley were reassigned to the Chilean border to prevent precursors being smuggled into Bolivia, leaving the Chapare checkpoint under the control of UMOPAR. According to one US field adviser, precursors flooded into the Chapare 'by the truck load'.

In the field, where fewer eyes are watching and the financial stakes are higher, corruption is predictably worse. Two or three days a month, police let the druglords land their planes unhindered in return for kickbacks. The days are arranged by traffickers who come into the base and talk with the *comandante*, according to a Leopard. 'The *narco* says "On such and such a day, I'm going to land my plane," and hands over 10,000 bucks.'

A 1988 report by Bolivia's Permanent Assembly of Human Rights described the process.

> On [the appointed] days the anti-narcotics police shut themselves in their barracks so that large-scale operations can be carried out. This curious system, called *cobertura* [cover], is known by the police, *campesinos* and the traffickers' intermediaries. On these days planes arrive in the region to buy paste and base and drugs are sold freely in every little shop and newspaper kiosk. When the days of 'cover' are over, UMOPAR enter the area, commit abuses, raze houses and rob the *campesinos* of their money and possessions.

With the US keeping an eye on them, the police, instead of staying in barracks during days of *cobertura*, now actively patrol other areas in order to appear busy and to distract the attention of their superiors and the DEA.

The police only seize the trafficker's drugs and property, like cars, Rolex watches and guns, if he is unable to pay them off. Alternatively, they may make a deal with the trafficker whereby they take all his assets but promise in return not to report him. The booty is then shared out among the police and a symbolic portion brought back to the base as proof that a raid has been carried out. 'We used to hide the stuff in the pockets of our uniforms,' says one former Leopard, called Jorge. 'Sometimes, if the traffickers hadn't finished making their drugs, the police ordered them to carry on until they had, then let the workers free in return for the finished paste or base.'

Officially, the confiscated property is stored in a large room at Chimoré headquarters where it is carefully recorded. Cocaine is then burned and assets handed over to the state. In practice, things do not always work out that way, as Jorge, who when at Chimoré was in charge of the dope store-room, recalls. 'I would steal two kilos at a time and resell them in Sinahota. I had to be careful though, as everything was written down.' Jorge also began to consume the cocaine under his protection, and claims he was joined regularly by fellow police officers. His addiction finally got him expelled.

Other confiscated goods, he claims, were hidden on the base, then shared out. 'When the Americans came to inspect, once a month, we hid all the stuff in the mountain and brought it back again when they'd gone.' It is disposed of in a number of different ways. In the case of luxury cars, police officers may keep a couple of Mercedes for personal use then use their connections to get the necessary papers to resell the others in sale rooms in Santa Cruz or Cochabamba. Dope is sold either back to the traffickers or disposed of on the black market. Often police prefer the second option in case an angry trafficker decides to betray him. In Chimoré, police officers sell cocaine through women who enter the base posing as lovers, market it in Sinahota, and bring back the money after taking a cut. In Cochabamba, police resell cocaine paste to street children whose addiction they foster in the hope of making bigger profits. Some, like Bismarck Barrientos, quit the police force to become full-time traffickers.

US equipment also provides a lucrative source of income. Grocers in Cochabamba, for instance, can be found selling US Meals Ready to Eat. Their contents, from peanut butter to vacuum-sealed ham and turkey loaf, must provide culinary surprises for many ordinary Bolivians. US-supplied vehicle spare parts, uniforms, boots and weapons are also resold and US-loaned trucks and Piranha river patrol boats used as commercial taxi services.

Since US agents moved into Chimoré in the late 1980s, corruption has become more sophisticated. However, as the DEA admits, it is still extremely rife and that if they left things would almost certainly go back to how they were before. Even in December and January, when DEA agents return to the US for their Christmas holidays, operations virtually grind to a standstill. But some progress has been made, according to one senior DEA agent:

> When we first arrived, corruption was so blatant we didn't even need informants. What we have now is 'workable corruption' as opposed to some countries where you really can't do anything. Here you can still do the job. Things are improving. A couple of years ago we couldn't even tell the UMOPAR guys where we were going on an op until we were airborne. Now we do. We plan and go out on ops together.

The force has been cleaned up in a range of ways, from training police officers in the US, giving them extra pay, to putting pressure on the Bolivian government to appoint non-corrupt officials to key posts. In mid-1991 the Bolivian government claimed it was totally restructuring the force after a high-ranking officer suspected of operating a chemical smuggling ring from Chile committed suicide. As evidence of their increased effectiveness

UMOPAR officers point to Operation *Atipasunchaj* ('We will win', in Quechua) in November 1990 which cleaned many traffickers from the Red Zone.

To many Bolivians, however, the US 'obsession' with corruption is hypocritical and fails to take account of its root cause, poverty. As one Chimoré officer put it:

> There's corruption in any country, Bolivia, the US, anywhere. But it's perhaps more understandable in Bolivia, where an officer earns 50 bucks a month and has eight children to support than in the US where he would earn well over 500. The *gringos* here can go to Cochabamba every 30 days and stay in a nice hotel with a swimming pool. We're stuck here day and night. We can't even afford to go to the village bar.

US criticism is seen as an unwarranted intrusion into the affairs of another country. 'How would the Americans feel,' asks the official, 'if we went to the US to investigate corruption there and published reports on it?' The US response to the problem has been to increase police numbers and reinforce them with the military. But most Bolivian police believe that, in the words of Oliver Cromwell, 'A few honest men are better than numbers.' They say the most effective way to tackle police corruption would be to reduce the number of UMOPAR so that the remaining ones can be paid decent salaries and become a professional and motivated force.

For police officers who do try to clean up, the obstacles are enormous. One officer, who asked not to be named, admits that his refusal to play the game has left his family far worse off than those of his colleagues. 'I've been a policeman 15 years, and only now am I buying my own apartment. I used to have a Mercedes but I had to sell it. On the days when it rains and I'm getting soaked waiting for a taxi I ask myself if it's worth it. But at least I have a clear conscience.' The other price he pays is isolation. If he knows about a trafficker he cannot tell anybody because he never knows to whom he is talking. He has few friends. In the evenings, instead of drinking with buddies in the local bar, he stays at home reading Spanish novels. His attitude astonished the traffickers.

> I am the *narcos'* enemy Number One because they know I won't take bribes. They don't even come near me. They know that if they do, I'll not only say No, but I'll chase them all over Bolivia. A few months ago a trafficker asked me to take a million dollars to allow him to land his plane and I immediately launched a raid against him.

Often, though, he says there is little point in catching traffickers because his actions are bound to be compromised further along the line.

> If I catch a big trafficker I can be sure that when he gets to gaol the judge or some government official will let him out a fortnight later. It makes a mockery of my work. It also puts my life in danger: the traffickers, once free again, send

me death threats. They send them to me, not to the Americans because they know that if they sent them to the Americans there'd be one hell of a response.

In fact, he says, politicians are often even more dangerous than traffickers because no-one knows who they are. 'At least with the traffickers you know where you stand. With politicians you don't: they don't admit outright that they are protecting the traffickers.' He believes one of the reasons police are so poorly paid is that the government does not want to support them. In Yacuiba, in eastern Bolivia, a patrol of narcotics police was actually locked out of its offices after the government failed to pay its rent for 11 months. Police raids are frequently compromised after government tip-offs, the officer claims, and seized assets which could be used to make the police more efficient are instead used to line the pockets and garages of government officials. 'The government says the drug war is going well or badly according to what it thinks will win it votes,' he says. 'But it doesn't really care. We have to rely on US supplies and help instead.'

ON 23 February 1990, a ten-man UMOPAR patrol drove into a village west of Isinuta. It was midnight, and their goal was to go in at first light to seize a large consignment of cocaine which two informants had told them about. Suddenly, the men came under a hail of automatic weapons fire while villagers blocked the road with burning tyres. The police leaped out of their trucks and moved in tactical formation through the houses. But the ambush was an expert one and heavy shooting ensued, during which the traffickers ran off with the drugs. One, a Colombian, shot at a police lieutenant with a 45-calibre submachine gun. The lieutenant fired back with his Korean-made M1 carbine but it failed to function and he died soon after UMOPAR's first casualty. When anti-drugs agents later inspected the carbines used by the patrol, they found four out of ten did not work. The dead man's rifle carried only two rounds of ammunition.

Two months later the US embassy delivered 50 M-16 rifles and began training on their use. Another 400 arrived later in the summer. 'It took the lieutenant's death to get us the M-16s,' says Colonel Vargas ruefully.

Antiquated equipment is one of the Leopards' largest obstacles. 'How can we compete with the traffickers when we have World War Two carbines which are falling apart, and they have the latest Israeli Galil assault rifles?' asks one. UMOPAR's ancient radio equipment too is unable to compete with the *narcos'* sophisticated Japanese-made equipment.

The traffickers, because of their vast financial resources, will always be several steps ahead. But large quantities of equipment, from uniforms, to weapons to aircraft, provided by the US are now enabling the police to go a little way to catching up. European governments, like Spain and Britain, have also chipped in, although their contribution remains minimal compared to that of the US. Britain, for example, has given the UMOPAR unit in Trinidad, Beni, three short-range VHF Racal radios, two long-range ones and a number of sniffer dogs. But this falls short of the 15 short-range and five long-range radios the commander of the base believes he needs. Spain has also donated large numbers of M-16s and other equipment.

Unlike US-provided aid, European equipment tends to have few strings attached, a fact welcomed by one police officer who resents his total dependence on The Embassy.

> We've been waiting nearly ten years for certain things but they've still not arrived. When they do arrive, they come with rigid conditions attached. Take the uniforms, for example. If my men's uniforms are getting old I have to go to the embassy and beg. The Americans make us show the old ones. If they think the uniforms are still wearable they make us take them back. When they give us new ones we have to return the old ones. It's humiliating. They give us one uniform a year. My men should have four, and four pairs of boots. Can you imagine going out into that boiling jungle every day in the same uniform? The men need to change their clothes when the uniform gets dirty but with only one they can't. It's the same with the boots. They wear out in two months. If the men go on wearing them they get fungal infections.
>
> Take the vehicles too. We have one vehicle for every 55 men. They're supposed to be replaced every two years, but they haven't been changed for four years. Often we don't even have enough petrol to run them. And guns. When we wanted US guns, it took three years to negotiate. The government said it was because they didn't want to upset the army. Why, then, did they accept the guns which were sent us by the Spaniards? When the Americans send things they have so many conditions. The Europeans and the Japanese are different; when they give us something, it's a real gift.

On a day-to-day level, relations between the Leopards and the Americans are good, although few DEA agents stay long enough for the Bolivians to remember their names. 'They all seem to be called Robert or Bill, so it's very confusing,' says Vargas. 'And their surnames are far too difficult. So the Leopards give them nicknames like Rambo, which are easier to remember.'

Higher up, though, friction is evident. The DEA team leader regales Vargas with bottles of whisky when he returns from rest and recuperation, but ultimately the *comandante* knows it is the DEA, not he, who call the shots. Officers on Vargas's level resent the fact that US military advisers at Chimoré are training Leopards when they have no knowledge of the local language or terrain. 'We know far more about law enforcement in Bolivia than they do,' says one officer. 'They can learn from us if they want, but there is little they can teach us.' They also resent the DEA's tendency, in the past at least, to plan most operations, and in some cases to keep them secret from the Bolivians. Many do not appreciate being forced to assume a subordinate role within their own country. 'You have to stand up to the Americans,' says one. 'If you show the slightest weakness, they trample all over you. I try to make it into a relationship between friends, that's to say, between two people on an equal footing. If you don't agree with something they suggest, you have to say No. You have to hang on tightly to your identity.'

A further cause of resentment is the US decision in 1989 to step up the role of the Bolivian army and to increase their resources at the expense of those given to the police. According to one official quoted by a US congressional report,[1] the disparity in resources was seen by UMOPAR as 'nothing short of a slap in the face'.

Policy makers in Washington believed the army was necessary to deal with traffickers whom they claimed were becoming increasingly violent. The army would support the police by providing extra resources and manpower.

Unfortunately, Bolivian history shows that the idea of the two bodies working together is totally fanciful. The Bolivian police and army have been at loggerheads ever since the 1952 revolution which attempted to curb the power of the army and strengthen that of the police. There is still no love lost between them. In one recent incident, for example, two policemen at Chimoré were nearly beaten to death by soldiers in the René Barrientos Military Barracks across the road. One fell into a coma and had to be taken to hospital in Santa Cruz. In another incident, recounted by a DEA source, a UMOPAR instructor was seized by soldiers in the barracks and was hung in the shower where they 'beat the hell out of him'. He would have died had a fellow UMOPAR officer not managed to rescue the man. As the source put it, 'If a military guy has a choice of killing a trafficker or a UMOPAR, he will kill the UMOPAR guy every time. They hate each other's guts.'

Bolivian police also feel strongly that the army is inappropriate for what is an intelligence and investigation operation. 'It may be that the US doesn't understand this,' says one. 'But you can't use tanks or bombs against the *narcos*. This is thick jungle. They call this a war on drugs, but it's not a real war; it's a low-intensity conflict. The reason the military want to get involved is to get nice uniforms and travel to the US.' Another police officer compares the respective roles of the police and the army with those of a surgeon and a butcher.

> Imagine both had to treat a man with a tumour in his arm. The butcher, when he comes to the arm, will cut it off. The surgeon, on the other hand, will cut out the tumour and sew up the wound: the man still keeps his arm. This is what I have to do as a policeman. I have to identify traffickers and get them out of society. But I can't wipe out everybody in the hope of finding just them.

5

Cocaine Coups:
The Military

ON Thursday 17 July 1980, Bolivians awoke to the news that the army's sixth division, headquartered in the jungle city of Trinidad, in the Beni, had rebelled and was calling for its organiser, a portly army chief called General Luis García Meza, to lead a 'national revolution' to save the country from 'communist extremists'. The 189th coup in Bolivia's 154 years of independence had begun.[1]

In La Paz, Bolivia's national trade union organisation, the COB, called an emergency meeting. Around 30 trade unionists, priests, politicians and human rights leaders hurried through the winter cold to the COB's humble second-floor headquarters on the city's main thoroughfare, the Prado. Among them was Marcelo Quiroga Santa Cruz, a lawyer and a socialist candidate in the recent general elections who had recently antagonised the military by calling for an investigation into human rights abuses under Banzer's dictatorship. On the other side of town, at the presidential palace, Lidia Gueiler, the interim president, led an emergency cabinet meeting.

At 10.30 a.m. news reached the COB that the main square in Santa Cruz had been taken by rebels and that military units in Cochabamba had joined the coup. The trade unionists had seen plenty of coups in their time and didn't take too much notice. 'Even then, we thought it was all a practice run,' recalls one of Quiroga's colleagues. 'We didn't take it too seriously.' Quiroga proposed a general strike. The idea was accepted and a strike call was immediately issued to radio stations and newspapers across the country.

Suddenly, at midday, the group heard gunfire. At first they assumed the firing was simply meant to intimidate. As the windows began to shatter, they realised this coup was different. They were under attack. The group huddled together on the floor to dodge the bullets pelting through the window. Moments later a couple of ambulances drew up outside the building. Around 30 hooded civilians climbed out, rushed up the stairs with automatic weapons and ordered everyone outside, leaders first.

'Get out of here, you sons of a bitch,' shouted one gunman.

'Don't shoot, we are unarmed,' said a priest as everyone put their hands on their heads. The killers appeared nervous, keen to get on with their job.

One spotted Quiroga. 'Look who's here,' he said smiling. As the group left the building, he ordered Quiroga to stay behind. Quiroga refused and tried to bolt, but the gunman pushed the others in front and sprayed him with machine-gun fire. He and two other friends died shortly afterwards.

The survivors were taken by jeep and ambulance (stolen by the military from the Bolivian Red Cross) to the headquarters of the joint chiefs of staff, where they were beaten and tortured. The women were raped. 'They threw us into the stables and forced us to spend the night in the dung. One thug tried to interrogate me about the COB's "armed group",' recalls Simón Reyes, a miners' union leader. 'Kill me if you want, you bastard,' I told him. 'He struck me on the back of my neck with his rifle and beat me till I was almost unconscious.'

Next morning at 6.00 they were taken to the offices of the secret police. 'We were crammed 20 to a cell, without food and living in our own excrement,' remembers Reyes. 'We were tortured by hooded paramilitaries with Italian or Argentine accents. I was beaten so brutally I thought I wouldn't survive. It was a month and a half before I received my first visit.'

The Italian and Argentine accents belonged to paramilitary thugs who had helped carry out the coup. The Italians were members of a gang of neo-Nazis led by Klaus Barbie, who had previously worked for Roberto Suárez. They worked with members of the Argentine military who had just carried out their own 'dirty war' across the border. The army chief, García Meza, hoped they would pass on their latest techniques in repression to the Bolivian military.

Keen to prevent mass resistance, which had thwarted previous coups, the military fanned out through the city in tanks and armoured personnel carriers, attacking pre-selected targets of potential civilian opposition. Vigorous steps were taken to crush the COB strike, and the Catholic radio station, Radio Fides, was quickly silenced. La Paz turned into a ghost town as a 9.00 p.m. to 7.00 a.m. curfew was imposed and anyone who disobeyed it shot on sight.

Meanwhile, several cabinet ministers of Gueiler's interim government had been arrested at the presidential palace and imprisoned in the army headquarters. Gueiler was taken to the presidential residence where she received a phone call from one of the coup leaders, Colonel Luis Arce Gómez.

'Señora,' he said, 'on the instructions of General García Meza, we order you to resign in favour of the armed forces.'

Gueiler slammed down the phone and decided to get out. But as she got to the door, she realised she was a prisoner. The guards, previously subservient, said coldly they had been told not to let her out.

The doorbell rang. Two previously loyal military generals, Reyes Villa and Waldo Bernal, were on the doorstep.

Bernal handed over a resignation document which had been drawn up at the army barracks. Gueiler threw it onto the table. 'How do you expect me to sign that?' she said. For several hours, the group thrashed things out with the help of the papal *nuncio* who had been called in to mediate. Realising that she had no choice but to sign, Gueiler called in her foreign minister.

'I'm going to give you a very hard and sad task,' she told him. 'I want you to reword this resignation and make it more dignified.'

The show began. Television cameras were wheeled into the drawing room, plus a journalist, Donald Zabala, whose face made clear that he was there against his will. Gueiler sat down, the foreign minister on one side, the *nuncio* on the other. Villa and Bernal hovered by the door.

'Sit down,' Gueiler invited them.

'No thanks,' muttered one.

Sobbing, Gueiler read her resignation.

THE 17 July had gone well for the coup leaders. By the end of the day the presidential palace and the university were under military control and every radio station apart from the army's had been silenced. Outside the capital only the miners' radios kept going for a few days until they too were destroyed. The armed forces, declared the military radio, had quit barracks 'for the dignity of Bolivia'. They rejected the results of general elections which had been held the previous month, and declared Congress 'unconstitutional'.

The next day García Meza swore in a military junta and a cabinet. He named a friend of his, Arce Gómez, as interior minister, and a man called Faustino Rico Toro as chief of intelligence. Sporadic resistance continued, despite the arrests of more than 500 people in the first 24 hours, but massive arrests over the next few days mopped up those who had not managed to reach a foreign embassy or go underground.

Having secured the capital, military units moved into the mines of the Andean highlands with tanks and heavy weapons. In August dozens of striking miners at Caracoles were butchered after they blockaded the roads in protest at the coup. Paramilitary and regular units moved through the countryside to pre-empt resistance from the peasantry. Some 'disappeared' after being slung down 1,000-foot ravines in the Yungas, east of La Paz.

By September, between 1,500 and 2,000 people had been detained, all without charge. They were treated like pigs, forced to sleep on wet floors with their hands and feet bound, or to eat food from plates onto which guards had urinated. Men were given electric shocks on their testicles after being stripped, and beaten all over with wooden clubs. One prisoner, Adela

Villamil, a member of the Women's Federation, reported being beaten with a horsewhip, tied up and left hanging by her wrists. Then for three days she was locked in a wooden box, with a small hole for air. One night six uniformed men raped her and her cell mate. At one point she was pinned to a table and an electric prod was thrust up her vagina. Other 'leftists' were exiled, banished to labour camps in the jungle, or hid in hotels or the basements of half-finished buildings in La Paz.

García Meza, now installed as president, made clear he was here to stay. 'I will stay as long as I have to to eliminate the Marxist cancer, be it five years, ten or twenty,' he declared. His views and methods were eerily similar to those of a friend of his called General Augusto Pinochet.

So began the most brutal, corrupt and vicious regime that Bolivia had ever seen.

GENERAL García Meza and his close friend Colonel Luis Arce Gómez shared two passions: a visceral hatred of 'communism' and a sideline in cocaine. Both knew the best way to satisfy both was to seize power.

García Meza, a thickset humourless bully known among his colleagues for his foul language and bellowing voice, was Bolivia's Noriega. Born into an army family in 1932 'Lucho', as he was nicknamed, was groomed from an early age to follow in the steps of his father, an army colonel. He was sent to the fashionable La Salle school in La Paz and then to the Colegio Militar where he met Arce Gómez. According to friends, at the age of 14 he was already talking about becoming president.

His first important promotion was to the position of army chief under the military dictatorship of Colonel Alberto Natusch in 1979, but he lost the job two weeks later when the regime was replaced by the interim civilian government of Gueiler, a distant relative of his. Halfway through her term in office, however, she reappointed him to the post, assuming that giving him power was the best way of keeping him quiet. It was her biggest mistake.

García Meza's bid for power was backed by Colonel Arce Gómez, a 'crude pot-bellied 50 year-old thug who enjoyed donning the dark glasses of a stage dictator'. Sophistication was not one of his assets and he had always been bottom of the class at the Military Academy in La Paz. His colleagues nicknamed him 'Opa Luis' (Simple Luis), or when they wanted to be polite, 'Lucho'. He also had an uncanny knack of rubbing people up the wrong way. He was expelled from the academy for trying to run away, and then again from his next establishment for mutinying against a presidential order appointing a new commander-in-chief of the army. The army booted him out for allegedly raping the daughter of a superior, and he took up as a society photographer for a national newspaper.

Reincorporated into the military under the military dictatorship of General Barrientos, Arce Gómez's break came in 1979 when he was appointed chief of military intelligence, or 'Section Two' as it was known, a position from which he quickly moved to take control of Bolivia's entire internal security machine. He did this in his own inimitable style by raiding the offices of the only rival intelligence organisation in Bolivia, the secret police. Arce Gómez held up officials at the Ministry of the Interior at machine-gun point and carried off the secret police records to the dreaded Section Two.[2] He installed wire taps on the telephones of hundreds of Bolivian politicians, military officers and trade unionists. Others were watched closely by military spies. 'I knew everything,' Arce Gómez boasted later. 'I knew exactly who was homosexual in the police. We controlled politicians' telephones too. We knew all their family problems, what kind of life their daughters and wives lived, whose daughters worked as prostitutes, whose wives were having affairs with their best friends. If I'd spoken lots of families would have fallen apart.'

Both men made no secret of their belief that democracy in Bolivia was 'premature' and could lead to political chaos. Worst of all, it could threaten the country's institutions, especially the military. 'Democracy hasn't yielded any positive results in this country,' García declared in a speech in 1980. 'Democracy has been confused with the behaviour of libertines.' Like Pinochet, García Meza believed democratic governments should leave it to the military to decide how it wanted to be run, and was outraged at Gueiler's insistence on appointing the military's high command. More galling still, Hernán Siles Zuazo, whom everyone expected would be elected president in June 1980, had hinted that this government might investigate 'wrong-doings' by the military under previous dictatorships.

Ignoring grunts of disapproval from other sectors of the army, the two men orchestrated a campaign of violence to topple the country's fragile democracy ahead of the June elections. Their main targets were left-wing and church groups, for example that producing the weekly magazine *Aquí*. In March 1980, the battered body of the magazine's editor, Father Luis Espinal, was found near a municipal slaughterhouse, apparently after he had run some stories about the death squads set up by Arce Gómez. In June, a vice-presidential candidate, Jaime Paz Zamora (now Bolivia's president) narrowly escaped death when the plane in which he was travelling crashed. The plane, it turned out, had been hired from a company owned by Arce Gómez.

The other thing on the two men's minds was cocaine. Both had seen the trade boom from a cottage industry to a multibillion-dollar business under General Banzer. By 1981 cocaine had become Bolivia's largest export, earning nearly four times as much as the country's second commodity, tin. They knew that control of the coke trade would give them unprecedented wealth and power. 'We are going to inundate the *gringos* with cocaine,' Arce Gómez reportedly told a colleague.

Arce Gómez was no stranger to the trade. Since the early 1970s he had combined a military career with a profitable sideline in drugs. In 1975 he set up an air taxi business to carry cocaine. By 1980 he operated eight aircraft. As head of Bolivia's security machine, Arce Gómez also owned all the narcotics files, stolen from the secret police. He also happened to be related to Roberto Suárez. As the 1980 elections had approached, Arce Gómez had been worried that a civilian government would clamp down on the cocaine trade and investigate his activities. The only way to stop that was to run the country and the industry himself.

To achieve his aims, Arce Gómez hired a man who had the ideal qualifications: Klaus Barbie, the ex-Nazi SS officer known as the 'Butcher of Lyons'. As Gestapo chief of the French city Lyons, he was accused of ordering the execution of 4000 French citizens, including the French resistance leader Jean Moulin, and sending 7000 to German death camps. Ironically, it was the CIA which had shielded Barbie from the French authorities and helped him escape to Bolivia after the war because of fears his capture might reveal the operations of the US Counter-Intelligence Corps for whom Barbie had worked in Europe. In Bolivia, Barbie had worked for Banzer's Interior Ministry in counter-intelligence; then, when Banzer had been ousted, he had acted as security consultant to Roberto Suárez. He therefore had an intimate knowledge both of Bolivia's cocaine trade and of its repressive apparatus. Under Banzer he had 'perfected' the interrogation methods used by Bolivian intelligence.[3] According to an Interior Ministry official, Barbie brought a subtler touch. 'The Bolivians used simply to beat people up. Under Barbie, they learned the use of techniques of electricity and the use of medical supervision to keep the suspect alive until they had finished with him.' Arce Gómez believed Barbie was the perfect man to train his paramilitary hit squads.

Arce Gómez later denied that his relationship with Barbie was a close one. But his version at the time was different. Introducing Barbie to a journalist in 1980, Arce Gómez said: 'This man is my teacher.' In 1981 he introduced Barbie to a military acquaintance as 'my great friend Don Klaus'.

Barbie recruited a band of young neo-Fascists and neo-Nazis whose views and methods were as uncompromising as his own. Known as the Fiancés of Death, the group included the Italian terrorists Stefano delle Chiaie (who had trained under the Chilean secret police), his friend Pier Luigi Pagliai, the young neo-Nazi Fiebelkorn, and Manfred Kuhlmann, a Rhodesian mercenary. Most had been trained by, and worked for, the Argentine Secret Service. In Bolivia they belonged to shady newly established organisations within the Interior Ministry which drilled Arce Gómez's paramilitary units. After hours they gathered at a German beerhall in Santa

Cruz, called the Club Bavaria, where they sang old Nazi battle songs and watched Second World War documentaries.

In early 1980 plans for the coup were almost ready. Barbie summoned his gang to their hide-out in Santa Cruz. The putsch, he said, was part of the world-wide fight against communism. 'The moment has come. We have to overthrow this government before Bolivia becomes another Cuba.'

The drug traffickers were delighted. Having been protected by a succession of military governments, they were getting increasingly nervous about the prospect of democracy. They were keen to set up a government of their own. In early 1980, Roberto Suárez convened a meeting at the Club Bavaria to which he invited Erwin Gasser, Barbie, and a well known trafficker. They offered García Meza $1.3 million to launch a coup, promising him vast profits afterwards. Their only condition was that Arce Gómez, with whom they had dealt for years, be made minister of the interior in charge of anti-narcotics operations.[4]

By April the coup leaders were so confident that they did not even bother to hide their intentions. The none-too-secret preparations prompted the new US ambassador Marvin Weissman publicly to warn García Meza and the military not to attempt a takeover. García Meza reacted with scorn, declaring Weissman *persona non grata* and even threatening his life, confident that once in office the US would offer him the same support it had given Banzer.

Eight weeks later, on 29 June 1980, democratic elections were held and won by Hernán Siles Zuazo, who headed the leftist Popular Democratic Union (UDP) party. He was due to take office in August. On 17 July García Meza and his friends decided to strike. For the first time in history, the $1,500 million-a-year cocaine trade had 'bought itself a government', remarked one US official. The *Miami Herald* called it the 'cocaine coup'.

Shortly after the coup, according to an internal memo by the DEA, which pulled out immediately after the takeover, the Santa Cruz drugs Mafia declared it was 'prepared to supply all the money that is needed by the new military government for a period of several months'.[5] Another report, by a contributor to the *New York Times*, recounted how a group of traffickers went to La Paz in the week after the coup to offer the government at least $70 million to help cover repayments on Bolivia's foreign debt which was creeping towards $3,000 million.[6]

At first, the cocaine generals took a percentage cut from the cocaine trade. Exporters were allegedly forced to pay a tax of $2,000 per kilo, providing the government with around $200 million a year. A trafficker who wished to take off in an aeroplane unhindered by the authorities paid up to $30,000 a time. Even owners of bales of coca leaf, worth $40, were forced to hand over a quarter.

Soon, García Meza and his cronies realised they could make greater profits if they concentrated production and squeezed out smaller cocaine manufacturers. This would leave a few big traffickers who could pay decent protection money and could be more easily controlled. Suppressing the small fry, the generals hoped, would also serve another purpose: to convince the US, which had severed diplomatic relations and withdrawn economic and military aid, that Bolivia was clamping down on drugs.

The benefits of the plan were spelt out in a Bolivian Defence Ministry report in December:[7]

> Even before initiating the campaign of concentration of production, you could collect, without difficulty, around $200 million annually, on the basis of a tax of $2,000 per kilo, which all the exporters were willing to pay, as a single tax. If we can guarantee all the industrial process and the suppression of the intermediaries, without prejudicing the interests of the peasant producers of the leaf, this sum could rise to $600 million annually.

According to one of the Fiancés, García Meza and Arce Gómez called Barbie, Fiebelkorn and two Fiancés to a meeting at the Ministry of the Interior to discuss the strategy. Arce Gómez handed Fiebelkorn a list of 140 smaller Santa Cruz dealers who were to be 'suppressed' by special paramilitary squads set up by Arce Gómez and Barbie. None of the big drug barons, including Suárez, was on the list.[8]

Using techniques borrowed from Argentina, the special paramilitary squads set up by Arce Gómez seized cocaine from traffickers who were not paying for protection and stored it in bank vaults. It was then redistributed to traffickers who were paying protection, like Suárez, or handed to the Ministry of the Interior which resold it. Some gang members exported cocaine to the US and Europe in exchange for weapons. Any property confiscated by the paramilitaries in the course of their operations, like houses, money, planes and cars, was considered a perk of the job which they were allowed to keep. In three months the Fiancés of Death reportedly seized 20 luxury cars and over $300,000 in cash.

Penalties for traffickers who did not play according to the rules were harsh. One of Fiebelkorn's admirers recalls: 'Everybody who was in the traffic had to pay 10 per cent to Arce in an office on the eighth floor of the Edificio Santa Cruz [in Santa Cruz]. Whoever didn't pay, died.' In the course of three months, 15 men in Santa Cruz who broke the rules paid with their lives.[9]

The man who made the richest pickings and who effectively ran the show was Arce Gómez, later dubbed by a CBS television Sixty Minutes programme in February 1981 as the 'Minister of Cocaine'. According to one Bolivian military source he was receiving $200,000 a week from the druglords. For one 240-pound shipment to the US in 1980, he got $40,000.[10] Soon he owned 11 planes, mansions in Santa Cruz and in La Paz, and a luxury *hacienda* with an airstrip.

US Senator Dennis De Concini, whose investigations provided the basis of the Sixty Minutes programme, claimed that Arce Gómez ran his own private processing and smuggling operation. One of his key linkmen with the US was a trafficker named Hernán Echeverría, now serving a five-year gaol sentence in the US, who liaised with Robbie Suárez Junior.

Other military officers were also cashing in. One named by De Concini was Hugo Echeverría, commander of the powerful Second Army Corps in Santa Cruz (no relation to Hernán). He was reportedly in overall charge of protection and transportation, and supervised the transport of cocaine from an international airfield to Venezuela, Colombia and the US. A Bolivian military official, called Rudy Landívar, who worked for him said later that Echeverría personally received 'masses' of protection money every day from the traffickers. 'At that time,' he told *El Mundo* newspaper in May 1988, 'both the Second Army Corps and the Rangers Regiment were almost taken over by drug trafficking, which is why they covered up the illicit situation that existed.'

Another Mafia member was Colonel Ariel Coca who had been made minister of education. Interior Ministry sources quoted by Sixty Minutes showed that Coca co-owned a huge jungle ranch on which air taxis landed and loaded up with cocaine. In 1979, the sources said, the pilot of a light aircraft which had been forced down in Panama had named Coca as the source of the 100 kilos that were found on board. The pilot was his brother-in-law.

Drug corruption filtered all the way down the armed forces. Many air force officers, for example, were unable to resist the temptation to carry a few kilos of cocaine on the side in return for huge rewards. 'Many air force officers retired and worked for the traffickers,' recalls one military source. 'We lost about 10 or 12 this way. They were paid $50,000 a trip to fly cocaine from Bolivia to Leticia in Colombia. Soon they got rich enough to buy their own planes.' For navy personnel too, it was all too easy to use their boats to ferry cocaine shipments.

Others worked as go-betweens, like Major Luis Cossío, commander of the military police battalion in La Paz. He was responsible for paying the Fiancés. According to one ex-member of the gang, Cossío brought $100,000 a month in cash to Fiebelkorn.

Another was a trafficker called José Abraham Baptista. He was a civilian police detective in Santa Cruz who had been assimilated into the army and promoted to second lieutenant. Baptista's job was to collect money from the *narcos* in his army office and to hand it over to his bosses, García Meza and Echeverría. He also supplied credentials to Barbie's gang of neo-Nazis so that they could pass as members of the Bolivian army.

But Baptista was dealing with fire and in October 1980 he got burnt. One day his contacts told him that five Colombians were arriving in Santa Cruz with $6 million to buy cocaine. Baptista found out which hotel they were staying in, murdered them and stole the money. He sent a cut to García Meza, but the general did not think it enough. He got on the phone to

Baptista's own squad of paramilitaries and told them to dispose of their leader. One October night, they killed him.

BY EARLY 1981 Bolivia's cocaine industry was clearly spiralling out of control. US officials estimated that Bolivia was producing four times more coca leaf than it could consume. Cocaine production had increased fivefold since García Meza had seized power. 'The export is getting out of control. Bolivia is growing more coca than coffee,' the DEA's Peter Bensing told Sixty Minutes. 'Lots of people are pulling up coffee and putting in coca. Business has never been better.' A narcotics specialist at the State Department was even more vocal, saying 'There is probably nothing short of communist revolution or nuclear obliteration that will stop [the boom].'[11]

Within Bolivia there was concern too, though not so much over drug trafficking as over the atrocities being carried out by paramilitary squads in the name of quashing 'subversion'. At the end of 1980, 150 political prisoners were still being held and around 100 had 'disappeared', according to Amnesty International. Some 1,500 Bolivians had been exiled. Millions of those who stayed at home had been cowed into terrified apathy following Arce Gómez's sinister remark, after introducing a new security law, that 'anyone who violates these laws had better walk with his will under his arm.'

The man Arce Gómez used to run his reign of terror was his former classmate and riding companion, a mustachioed colonel called Rico Toro who had taken over as army intelligence chief. 'He is a good friend, my best friend,' Arce Gómez said of him in 1991.[12] Nicknamed 'the magician' because of his skill at making leftists 'disappear', Rico Toro's reputation as an anti-communist hardliner went back to 1967 when he had taken part in the campaign against Che Guevara. A couple of years later he had been accused of being responsible for a plane crash that had killed the former President Barrientos, but had been saved from having to go to gaol by the arrival in power of General Banzer, who banished him to a remote posting on the border. But in 1978 Rico Toro was restored to respectability with a posting as military attaché in Washington. He was also believed to be responsible for setting up a Masonic lodge known as the 'Black Eagles' whose aim was to 'rule Bolivia for 20 years, killing some 2,000 leftists'. Membership of the lodge was a passport to key military posts.

In early 1981, however, even the middle classes had been alienated after a particularly gruesome attack. At 6.00 p.m. on 15 January around 20 paramilitaries had surrounded a house in the Calle Harrington in the exclusive Sopocachi district of La Paz where nine leaders of the left-wing Movimiento de la Izquierda Revolucionaria (MIR) party were meeting. Realising the house was surrounded, one of the deputies went to a window and shouted 'We're unarmed. Don't shoot.' The gunmen responded with a burst of machine-gun fire. They proceeded to torture and kill all but one of them, who, according to one report, saved her life by hiding under a bed. The official version was that security forces had disrupted a meeting of 'subversive delinquents'.

Many members of the military, some of whom had originally supported the coup in the belief that it was a legitimate attempt to save the armed forces from assault by leftist politicians and trade unionists, were repelled by the atrocities being carried out by the armed forces, sometimes even against their own men, and the appalling image the cocaine generals were giving the country. Hundreds of conscripts deserted. At one point the government was so desperate for recruits it resorted to seizing youths attending weekend football matches.

Even the traffickers became disgruntled. They found the protection money demanded by government officials excessive and the squads' methods distasteful. Also, the army traffickers had hit the independent dealers so badly that the supplies on which the big kingpins depended were drying up.

The cocaine generals became worried. The paramilitary squads seemed to have taken power into their own hands and were running amok. Internationally Bolivia was being outlawed, largely because of the attitude of the US which had made it clear that it would have no truck with a regime which so openly dealt in cocaine. Even newly elected President Ronald Reagan, whom García Meza had hoped would be more sympathetic to the regime, left Bolivia in the cold.

In November 1980, Arce Gómez went on a fence-mending visit to Washington at the invitation of the extreme right-winger Jesse Helms. But the trip turned into a fiasco after he tried to lay a wreath on the tomb of the unknown soldier at Arlington Cemetery. Officials made it clear his offering would not be welcome but Arce Gómez, unused to being told No, jumped over the fence and deposited a wreath all the same, to the dismay of the tomb's guard of honour. Arce Gómez claims the visit was partly to see the DEA, but the DEA refused to see him.

The last straw came in February 1981 when CBS broadcast its devastating Sixty Minutes programme, accusing Arce Gómez of being Bolivia's Number One trafficker.

García Meza realised he had to act. In late February, just a few days before the Sixty Minutes programme was aired, he quietly eased Arce Gómez out of his job as minister of the interior and made him head of the military academy, an appointment which enraged many members of the armed forces. Ariel Coca was sacked too. General Banzer, who had good links with the US and who was a friend of García Meza, was dispatched to Washington to try to persuade State Department officials to normalise relations. García Meza set up an army-led body called the National Council for the Fight Against Drug Trafficking, which he hoped would open the way for the DEA to return to Bolivia.

On 1 April 1981, García Meza attended the weekly meeting of his general staff and summoned Colonel Gary Prado Salmón, a rebel officer who commanded strong support inside the armed forces and at the time held the post of G6, in charge of education.

'I'm sending you to be head of the Eighth Division in Santa Cruz,' García Meza told him.

'Do you realise if you do I will gaol those [neo-Nazi] thugs?' Prado asked.

'You have my support,' replied García Meza. By 6.00 p.m. that same day, Prado had taken up his new post.

His first job was to clean out the Fiancés of Death. Fiebelkorn was paid off and told to pack his bags and leave the country immediately. 'His house was full of Nazi paraphernalia. There was a portrait of Hitler on the wall,' recalls Prado. Fiebelkorn and other members of the group headed for Brazil where they were arrested for carrying a 'going home present' of three kilos of cocaine. Some neo-Nazis joined the ranks of the dozen or so rebel military officers who were plotting a coup to get rid of García Meza. Others informed on traffickers like Suárez, whom they claimed had never paid their wages when they worked for him as bodyguards, in return for cash.

Barbie was forced out of Cochabamba but was not expelled from the country. Instead, he moved to La Paz where he led a low-key existence under the name of Herr Altmann. He would often be seen crouched over a cup of coffee in Café La Paz, a few blocks from the US embassy. Finally, in 1983 he was extradited to France, where he was convicted in 1987 for 'crimes against humanity' and sentenced to life imprisonment. He died of cancer in 1991.

The next task was to clamp down on the drug traffickers, particularly the Big Five (including Suárez) whose capture the DEA had demanded as a condition for recommencing operations in Bolivia. But progress was slight. Suárez, whose operations had already been seriously squeezed by the uniformed druglords, was furious. He went to García Meza and ordered the lifting of the purge. García Meza agreed but said it would cost Suárez $50 million. Suárez paid up and the crack-down ended abruptly, but he never forgot the arrogance.

THE regime was in trouble. Government corruption did not stop at cocaine but had seeped into other traditional areas too. In May 1981 a scandal was uncovered which revealed that García Meza and his cronies were openly looting the country in much the same way as Ferdinand Marcos had in the Philippines. García Meza and two other commanders, it turned out, had entered into a private agreement with a Brazilian firm for the mining and commercialisation of semi-precious stones from public lands at a site called La Gaiba.

García Meza's attempts to impress Washington had failed so miserably that he gave up. In a characteristic fit of rage, he declared that the armed forces were ceasing their operations 'because of the poor reception given to their efforts by the consuming countries' — a scarcely veiled reference to the US, which was still refusing to normalise relations.

Meanwhile pressure from other military factions was mounting. Coup rumours were rife. Officers loyal to Banzer, to Natusch and to Prado were all making schemes to oust the government. On 3 August supporters of Natusch and Prado jointly launched a coup from Santa Cruz, backed enthusiastically by *cruceños*. After mediation by the church, García Meza agreed to resign. By 4 August he and his wife Olga had packed their bags and moved out of the presidential palace. The world's most notorious drug-running regime had come to an end.

JUST over one year later, in October 1982, President Siles Zuazo finally returned the country to civilian rule, two years late. García Meza, now living a life of discreet luxury at his mansions in Cochabamba and La Paz, decided to commiserate the day of his inauguration by attending a horse-jumping competition at the Equestrian Club in Santa Cruz. There he bumped into his old friend General Prado, also a keen horseman. Prado recalls the meeting:

> We got chatting. After the competition I invited him to my house. We sat there drinking right until the early hours of the morning. The more we drank the more open we became. I told him what I thought of his regime. 'You did some awful things,' I said. 'You shouldn't have got involved in drug trafficking. And you shouldn't have abused human rights like that.' He just listened. He finally left for his hotel at about 4.00 a.m. *'Hasta mañana,'* he said. When I got up the next morning, García Meza had gone. He left no explanation. It later turned out he had taken the first plane out of Bolivia to Buenos Aires.

García Meza knew what was coming. Four years later, on 7 April 1986, now sacked from the armed forces, he was summoned to appear before the Supreme Court of Justice in the picturesque Andean city of Sucre on eight sets of charges ranging from violation of the Constitution and sedition, to killing and torturing opponents. Proceedings had been initiated against García Meza and 54 of his collaborators two years earlier and the first stage of the trial carried out by Congress. García Meza was not the only one in the dock: Bolivia's justice system and more than a few politicians' reputations were on trial too. The press called it the Trial of the Century.

Dressed in plain clothes and flanked by a platoon of security guards, García Meza walked into the Sucre court through the presidential entrance and sat down solemnly in the defendant's box, deaf to the yells of the hundreds of students, workers and widows who had gathered outside the court to demand justice.

His defence was predictable: the coup, he said, had been an institutional decision by the armed forces. Anyone who disagreed with his opinions he dismissed as a communist. But when it came to awkward details, the ex-dictator was struck by amnesia. 'I can't remember, your honour', 'I don't know', 'I'm not aware of that' he said time and time again.

Meanwhile, García Meza was living peacefully with his wife and two male servants in a beautiful house from where he could look out onto the terracotta roofs of Sucre's whitewashed colonial houses and the dramatic mountains beyond. Wandering along the city's cobbled streets, he would sometimes bump into Juán del Granado, the courageous young lawyer who was prosecuting on behalf of García Meza's victims. Del Granado would be on foot, García Meza in his jeep. But García Meza had little to worry about. No-one in the government was particularly bothered with the trial. In Sucre he had plenty of influential friends in the military who would see that nothing happened to him, and the townspeople still treated him more like a respectable *señor* than a criminal. Some had even proposed him as town mayor, clearly impressed by the frequency with which he threw parties for them. Even local journalists seemed far more interested in his social activities than the trial. With luck his lawyers would draw out the process for years. The Trial of the Century was rapidly turning into a Century of a Trial.

In his spare time, of which he had plenty, García Meza rode his thoroughbred horses, visited the Union Club for a game of dice, or worked on his memoirs which he had titled *Experiences of a Dictator*. Oddly, when it came to writing memoirs which he would use against his enemies, the forgetful dictator suddenly became remarkably lucid.

In January 1988, however, a new charge was brought against him. He was accused of stealing the diaries of Che Guevara and selling them illegally to Sotheby's in London. The ex-dictator knew that this time he could not get off so lightly, especially as the Americans were putting strong pressure on the government to imprison him. Fearing García Meza would be threatened if he went to gaol, his wife Olga forced him to go into hiding, where he still is.

This would be impossible without high-level protection from the police and military and government officials. Many suspect that García Meza's chief protector is General Banzer, who is known to have paid him a night-time visit a few days before the coup. 'Military men stick together,' says one prominent MNR politician. 'Banzer is extremely worried that unless he protects him, García Meza might publish his memoirs which could say some very damaging things.' Banzer may also fear that once García Meza's case is closed, investigators could move onto him and his bloody dictatorship. Others believe Rico Toro is hiding the former dictator on one of his ranches.

Government officials are quite open about having seen García Meza and his family at barbecues, restaurants and parties. In 1991 General Emilio Lanza crossed paths with Olga at Santa Cruz airport. She reportedly insulted him, still bitter about attempts by Lanza and other military officers to oust her husband when he was in power. Oddly, although García Meza is still being hunted as a criminal and although he was expelled from the armed forces, the government is still paying him a military pension. According to newspaper reports, the former dictator gets around $350 a month, collected by his wife. Meanwhile his trial drags on. No-one in the government seems to want to speed it up. As one official put it, 'No-one wants the burden of having a prisoner like García Meza.'

ARCE Gómez did not have such luck. One Sunday in December 1989, the former strong man, clad in T-shirt and shorts, was preparing a lunchtime *asado* (barbecue roast) with his wife and his mother at their house just outside Santa Cruz. At one o'clock a group of around 50 men in civilian clothes, but heavily armed, arrived at the gate. The men, a mixture of Leopards and Interior Ministry officials, had come to arrest him. For once, Arce Gómez had not been warned.

For the previous seven years, Arce Gómez, now a podgy silver-haired 51, had been in hiding. In 1982 he had fled to Buenos Aires where he gave the military government a hand in running its death squads in return for asylum. In 1983 he was arrested after being indicted along with 17 others by a Miami federal grand jury and charged with two counts of conspiring to import and distribute cocaine in South Florida. Two weeks later, though, he was set free on a technicality and fled to Paraguay. More recently there had been rumours that Arce Gómez had been spotted in the Beni but nothing ever came of them. By 1989, facing growing pressure from the US, the Bolivian authorities had decided it was time to act.

Still in his shorts, Arce Gómez was whisked off to Santa Cruz airport and bundled on to a US air force plane to Miami. After the García Meza fiasco, Washington was not taking any chances.

The seizure actually amounted to a kidnapping since no drug trafficking extradition treaty exists between the US and Bolivia. Or rather it does exist but is so antiquated as to be useless. It dates from 1900 when the US was hunting Butch Cassidy. But cocaine not being one of Cassidy's specialities, the treaty did not cover drug trafficking. 'Trying to use the 1900 treaty is like driving a horse and buggy on a five-lane interstate highway. It just isn't up to coping with the modern day,' says a US official in La Paz. Over the past few years Washington has made intensive efforts to urge Bolivia to sign a new extradition treaty but La Paz, having observed the row over extradition in Colombia, clearly considers it a political hot potato. Instead, it argues that US requests for extradition could be covered by a 1988 Vienna trafficking convention. But the US dislikes the convention since it makes extradition discretionary rather than mandatory. In 1991, the Bolivian government followed Bogotá's example by passing a decree which barred traffickers from being extradited provided they surrendered within 120 days. Seven major traffickers gave themselves up under the amnesty, but Washington still saw it as a severe blow to its drug policy.

In 1989, the US had few worries about the illegality of Arce Gómez's deportation. 'Bolivia set a splendid example of using unconventional tactics against accused drug traffickers,' wrote the *Miami Herald* in an editorial. In Bolivia, however, it sparked uproar. Critics on the left argued that it under-mined Bolivia's sovereignty and set a dangerous precedent in that it gave a free rein to DEA secret activities. They believed Arce Gómez should have first appeared before the Bolivian courts to answer human rights charges and were worried that his extradition would deprive García Meza's trial of a key defendant. Others believed it was justified given the feeble state of Bolivia's justice system. Among these was President Jaime Paz Zamora who declared he had decided to allow Arce Gómez's seizure because of the 'terrible weaknesses and the terrible immorality which plagues our judicial system'. Only three days earlier, in fact, another drug trafficker had walked out of gaol on a legal technicality. Although Paz's backing for the US action resulted from US pressure, universal hatred for Arce Gómez meant he was backed by a large section of the population.

EIGHT years after his antics in Arlington Cemetery, Arce Gómez was back in the US. Only this time he was not interior minister but a common drug criminal. Inside Miami's Federal Correction Centre, he was imprisoned in the maximum security section, where another, even better known trafficker was also locked up: Manuel Noriega. The high security surrounding him is not so much to protect society from him as to protect him from society. 'The problem is the people who testify against each other,' says a prison guard. 'There's so much hatred and bitterness that someone could easily try to get rid of him.' Arce Gómez has two guards wherever he goes.

Unlike Noriega, Arce Gómez was tried within the year. The trial lasted a month, but it took the jury only two hours to reach the verdict: guilty of conspiring to import cocaine and guilty of possession with intent to distribute it. He stood expressionless as he heard a court clerk read the jury's decision.

Arce Gómez's lawyer argued it was unfair to try him 5,000 miles from home, without the benefit of key witnesses. 'What we have witnessed here is not just a trial but a public whipping,' he declared. The defence rested on two main arguments: first, that Arce Gómez had only protected Bolivian drug traffickers in the hope of obtaining information on bigger foreign ones in order to impress the DEA; second, that Arce Gómez's arrest was equivalent to a kidnapping.

The jury was also unimpressed by the attempts of the defence to portray Arce Gómez as an elderly and inoffensive family man by dragging his relatives to court, including his frail 75-year-old mother. Choleric outbursts from the defendant revealed that the savage beast within him was far from dead. At one point he even yelled at his lawyer to shut up. In March 1991 Arce Gómez was given 30 years.

His military uniform exchanged for the green standard prison issue, the former strong man cuts a pathetic figure. The intelligence chief who could once listen in on every Bolivian politician now has his own telephone conversations monitored. Not that he receives many calls. The only people who keep in touch with him now are his lawyer and his family. 'Nobody has been to visit me,' he told the Bolivian journalist Lupe Andrade in April 1991,[13] 'not even my friend Rico Toro'. He spends his days lifting weights to build up his biceps, making pillow cases to earn pocket money, and writing his memoirs.

'I don't regret anything,' Arce Gómez told Andrade from the tiny bare cell he shares with a huge Cuban. 'I am completely innocent, I have never killed anybody.' Did he feel angry or upset? 'No. I'm a military man, I am used to anything. Revenge doesn't surprise me, I'm a hard man. To make me cry, it has to be something really big. It's when I feel impotent that I cry.'

ALTHOUGH by the end of 1981 García Meza and Arce Gómez were gone, the military's links with drug trafficking did not disappear overnight. When the military retreated to barracks in 1982 with the election of President Hernán Siles Zuazo the ties begin to weaken. But in the areas where cocaine was grown and manufactured, corruption remained, and remains, endemic. Like the Leopards, the military compete for postings in the Chapare and the Beni, in which they can expect huge payoffs for looking the other way.

The force traditionally the most prone to corruption is the Bolivian navy, whose work consists of monitoring jungle rivers in areas so remote it is impossible to keep tabs on their activities. All too often, navy personnel are found transporting the cocaine they are meant to be seizing.

The power of the traffickers makes investigative journalism virtually impossible. But in 1988 a journalist called Wilson García, of the Cochabamba newspaper *Los Tiempos*, decided to probe. He found that in many cases the druglords and the navy were the same thing.[14]

In September 1986, he reported, a Leopard on duty at the checkpoint outside the UMOPAR base at Chimoré stopped a convoy of cars: a military jeep, a Land Cruiser and a Toyota. Ignoring assurances by the uniformed driver of the jeep that the cargo was food supplies for the navy, the Leopard, who had been tipped off by the DEA, discovered that the 'food supplies' consisted of over a tonne of cocaine base. On being questioned, the driver of the jeep admitted that the cocaine was destined for the Centro de Operaciones Especiales (COE) (Centre for Special Operations), a naval base in Puerto Villarroel, half an hour's drive from Chimoré. From there it would be taken by boat to labs in the Beni. Oddly, García found that the driver's links with the navy were not even mentioned in the eventual official reports on the seizure.

When García dug further he discovered that navy personnel at the COE were running drugs in a big way. The unit's commander, naval lieutenant Edgar Zalles, arranged for cocaine to be collected from villages in the Chapare. It was processed inside a naval shipyard, under the supervision of a lieutenant called Max Galdo, two kilometres from the base. The semi-processed cocaine was then sent up-river to Santa Ana. Galdo, now retired, had been passing intelligence information to the traffickers for years.

In October 1985, officers at the base threw a party to which they invited Luis Fernando Roca, Techo de Paja's brother. He was welcomed by Zalles and departed in his private plane the next day accompanied by the naval lieutenant's brother.

García quoted another official who described what happened to the cocaine money:

> On at least five occasions, the deputy to the rear admiral... came to our base on the pretext of buying wood, which he never did. I then found out that he had been sent from La Paz to pick up money from the base. Once Zalles sent two of his men to Chimoré and they came back with thousands of dollars two days after the man from La Paz had arrived. Once I walked into Zalles's room just as he was handing over between $8,000 and $10,000. That night the rear admiral's deputy left for La Paz.

Needless to say none of these details ever came out in the official reports which were revealed when navy personnel were dismissed.

Since 1988 the Bolivian navy has been taking an active part in the 'war against drugs' by carrying out riverine drug control operations and ferrying UMOPAR troops to remote areas. Not surprisingly, contact with drugs and traffickers has left it not less but more corrupt. When, for example, in June 1989, the DEA and UMOPAR mounted a night assault on Santa Ana to try to arrest the trafficker Hugo Rivero, their helicopters were fired on not by drug traffickers but by the Bolivian navy detachment in the town! Navy personnel are regularly spotted partying with traffickers in Santa Ana. Often corruption occurs because naval officers are posted in their home towns where traffickers may be relatives.

Corruption in the air force, whose pilots since 1983 have been used to flying helicopters carrying UMOPAR, is also rife. Air raids are frequently compromised by air force personnel, many of whom moonlight for the traffickers.

The other force, the army, has been mainly excluded from the drugs fight, largely because of its gruesome past. It has contributed only in small ways like manning border posts to control the import of precursor chemicals. But during the past few years, pressures have built up for greater army involvement. In April 1991 the first units were instructed by US Special Forces in fighting drugs. But many, including the military itself, fear this will have disastrous consequences, including corruption on a scale even worse than that in the air force and navy.

Some pressures come from inside the military. Historically there has always been bitter rivalry between the military and the police, and the war on drugs has made things much worse. High-ranking officers were furious that the police were getting all the state-of-the-art equipment, training and funding from the US government at a time when the military's own budget was being slashed. In 1989 a group of senior Bolivian army officers was so angry about the training of UMOPAR personnel at the US army's School for the Americas at Fort Benning, Georgia, that it sent a letter to the US embassy saying it would withdraw its own trainees if the Americans did not send the policemen home. By 1990 relations had reportedly got so bad that many Bolivian army officials refused to speak to UMOPAR officers when they met. 'We are badly equipped and trained compared to the police,' said an army general in an interview in 1991. 'Survival is the major reason we want to join in the war against drugs. In a sense we want to justify our existence. Our mission is to fight wars, we want to show the people that we can do that.'

The army, he claimed, would counterbalance the corruption of the police and restore law and order. 'Seeing how corrupt the police are, people have lost faith in them. Often I get calls from people asking for protection from the police. How often do you see policemen in gaol for corruption? Never. People want the army to restore moral principles.'

These rivalries and needs have been deftly exploited by the US which, seeing that its 'war on drugs' was getting nowhere, decided the only solution was to turn it into a real war using proxy US-trained native forces. It therefore promised the Bolivian army substantial military aid on one condition: that it became involved in counter-narcotics operations to tackle the 'internal security threat' posed by the traffickers. In May 1990 the US and Bolivian governments signed an agreement under which the US promised the military $33.7 million in aid: a sixfold increase from 1989's levels. In return, Bolivia would deploy two light infantry battalions and one engineer battalion against the traffickers (a total of around 1,500 men). Though US officials denied the link, according to US congressman Peter Kostmayer, Bolivia was told that US economic aid would be cut off if it did not accept the military aid.

Inside Bolivia, the agreement unleashed a furore. The Bolivian government realised it was so sensitive that it tried to keep it secret, and news of the accord did not reach the Bolivian press until ten days later when Antonio Araníbar, a leftist politician, heard about it during a private visit to Washington. Once the news was public, the government was forced to backtrack. The army, it said, would only become involved in fighting drugs if the president believed the police were unable to cope. Government officials, privately repelled by the idea of involving the army but desperate not to lose US aid, dreamed up alternative ways the army could be usefully employed. One of their more bizarre suggestions was to use it to set up environmental protection units that would enforce laws against pollution and deforestation.

Politicians of all ideological colours, trade unionists, church leaders and even military officers were, for once, united in opposing the involvement of the army which they feared would lead to a 'Colombianisation' of the drugs war. American officials argued that soldiers were necessary to curb the increasing violence of the drug traffickers, but most Bolivians believed their involvement would cause, not resolve, bloody conflicts between young conscripts and peasants. Violence would simply create more violence. If, as many feared, the army entered the Chapare, the consequences could be catastrophic.

People's other fear was that by rearming and training the military, the US would unwittingly prompt it to grab power yet again, possibly using the fight against drugs as a pretext. This was no idle threat in a country which has had more coups than years of independence and where soldiers in barracks have always kept half an eye on the presidential palace.

US plans, said one Bolivian diplomat in Washington, 'could provide a direct challenge to democracy'.[15] By encouraging the army to fight drugs, US policy implies that the military are better qualified than civilians to maintain public order. Washington could be undermining the very democracies it claims to support, and with no guarantee that the cocaine trade will be destroyed.

As those with memories longer than the three-year span of most US diplomats in La Paz can recall, American infusions of aid for the military had already prompted them to take power 35 years earlier. Almost immediately after Bolivia's 1952 social revolution had replaced the over-powerful army with civilian militias, the civilian government of Paz Estenssoro faced overwhelming pressures from the US to rearm. A strong military, Washington believed, was the only way to prevent the spread of communism and another Cuba. In return it promised substantial economic aid.

The Bolivian government, already weakened by factional squabbles, reluctantly agreed. Bolivia was soon to pay the price: in 1964 General René Barrientos seized power, and the military remained in power uninterrupted for the next 18 years. In the late 1960s, the US gave them injections of aid to combat 'communist' threats like Che Guevara. Ironically it was the same military who became the country's biggest drug runners.

During the 1980s Bolivia followed a regional trend towards civilian democracy. None the less the military has remained a potent force and, given Bolivia's past history, it would be irrational to believe that it is confined to the barracks for good. As Andean expert Donald Mabry testified to the US Congress, 'We may be seeing an aberration right now to see a civilian government.'

Many military and police personnel who were associated with the García Meza regime are still in office. As social conflict increases (as a result of repressive anti-drug policies and economic crisis) the temptation for the military to 'save' the nation may become irresistible. 'It only needs one man to take advantage of the situation,' says General Lucio Añez, former head of the Special Force for the Fight Against Drug Trafficking. 'Involving the army could endanger our democracy which has cost us so much to achieve.'

US officials, on the other hand, contend that appeasing the military with increased aid is the best way of stopping them staging a coup. Melvyn Levitsky, the US assistant secretary for International Narcotics Affairs, for example, declared that the military is 'far more likely to take a constructive approach if actively engaged in the drug war, as opposed to being left to criticise civilian efforts from the sidelines'. Another US official in La Paz declared 'There is a danger in strengthening the police at the expense of the army. Rivalry between the two agencies could be destabilising.' He sought to reassure sceptics by saying that he saw no anti-democratic tendencies within the army.[16] Another claimed 'There is more to coups than weapons. A few new rifles or trucks won't make any difference.'

Another Bolivian concern is that once in contact with drugs, the army will become as corrupt as it was under García Meza. According to some military sources, the prospect of huge payoffs is one of the main reasons why the army wants to become involved in the war on drugs. Like the Leopards, army officers see a stint in a drug zone as the chance to make the fortune of a lifetime. One US official in La Paz claims the army is 'very sensitive about corruption' and will make sure it does not occur by rotating its officers. But senior army officials like General Lucio Añez are not convinced. 'It could affect the army's prestige. This has taken years to recover after the García Meza regime. Only one member needs to have a problem and the whole institution becomes tainted. Involvement by the army will open up old wounds.' The dangers are recognised by one experienced DEA official in La Paz who admits the decision to involve the army is born more of Washington's desperation at losing the drugs war than of rational thinking. 'It's the biggest goddam mistake we've ever made,' he says. 'We're opening a box here we will have a lot of trouble closing. You 'aint seen corruption till you've seen the military involved in fighting drugs.'

Critics also fear that, with their new powers, some of the military might demonstrate the same kind of contempt for human rights as they had shown under García Meza. But Washington has another view. Involvement in the drugs war will, on the contrary, improve the army's image, some officials claim. 'An impoverished, poorly trained and equipped military, unable to feed its troops, is far more susceptible to corruption and human rights abuses,' declared Levitsky. The US, he promised, would 'work with the Andean militaries to eliminate human rights abuses.' But, he added, even if the military did commit some excesses, violence by 'subversives' and drug traffickers was a far greater threat to democracy.

> We oppose the[se] abuses [of Andean militaries] as a matter of national policy and always will. But we should not succumb to the notion of downtrodden peasant masses protesting in arms against social injustice, nor depict organisations like the Sendero Luminoso of Peru... as champions of human rights.... It is this violence, in conjunction with the narco-traffickers, that has regional democracy under assault.[17]

Another worry is that the army will be used as a scapegoat when the war on drugs fails. 'It's a big headache,' said one general. 'Once we are involved, they will be able to blame us if we fail. This will damage the image of our institution.' It could also prompt disgruntled army officers to launch a coup. The general adds that army efforts to thwart the traffickers have little chance of success as long as politicians are totally uninterested. 'We could succeed if there was a real will to destroy the drug trade. But if we did destroy it, it would affect the interests of a lot of people, from bankers to politicians, both in Bolivia and abroad. So what's the point of making the effort?'

As discussions about army involvement continued, many of the military themselves were becoming disillusioned over the one thing that had enticed them into the drugs fray: the promise of military hardware. 'We'll enter Mr Bush's show,' says one army general bitterly,

> but in return we want better pay and equipment. Instead of giving us the military aid in cash and allowing us to decide how we need to spend it, they bring us Vietnam leftovers, things which aren't any use any more, just as they dumped World War Two stuff on us in the 1950s. Bolivia is becoming a cemetery for old vehicles.

Since spare parts of this hardware can only be found in the US, Bolivia is forced to be dependent on the US, he says. Bolivia ends up with two types of incompatible hardware: US antiques and modern weaponry bought by Bolivia or donated by European countries. 'The Americans work like the traffickers. They offer the first snort of cocaine free. Then you're addicted,' the general says. He would prefer to be given free use of US military aid, which he says would enable him to arm and equip his troops properly.

Many Bolivians, including members of the military, believe fighting drugs is a law enforcement job, not a military one. The role of the military is to eliminate an external enemy, not to investigate and arrest criminals. 'The police have been trained to carry out law enforcement and are now very well prepared,' says a military source. 'Why drag in the army?' A more practical solution, he suggests, might be to strengthen Bolivia's law enforcement agencies and judicial systems so that they can do their job effectively.

On a practical level, it is difficult to see how the army would tackle the drug traffickers. The traffickers are not grouped neatly into an army, but are individuals who, as in Vietnam, are spread over a vast area, much of it impenetrable jungle. 'Trafficking networks are spread into all sorts of corners where they cannot be detected or eliminated by M-16s,' says Añez. Also, given the traffickers' vast resources, however many weapons or men the security forces have, the druglords will always have more. 'If we double our anti-drug forces, they can increase them tenfold. There will always be a huge distance between us and them,' says Añez.

What exactly the army is supposed to do remains a mystery. 'We still don't know where we are going or what we are going to do,' said a frustrated General Emilio Lanza, commander of Santa Cruz's Eighth Division, the division nearest the Chapare, in April 1991. One suggestion is that the army will be used to monitor Bolivia's porous jungle borders, currently guarded by a mere 100 men, for imports of precursor chemicals. But how a few hundred impoverished army troops would be prevented from succumbing to huge payoffs from traffickers and how they would control a border several thousand miles long is a mystery. Another suggestion is for the army to surround the Chapare, so that police could round up traffickers inside the cordon. In theory they could be used too to surround towns like Santa Ana which, until June 1991, were totally controlled by traffickers, while police carry out raids. US officials also stress that, as in the Barrientos days, the army will carry out civic action projects, like building roads, bridges and medical posts, aimed at winning hearts and minds and improving its public image. Critics on the left, however, believe these activities should be carried out by civilians, not soldiers.

US and Bolivian officials have also got no nearer to explaining how the army will be persuaded to cooperate with UMOPAR. In early 1990 the chief of the armed forces reacted furiously to the suggestion by the head of police that the Special Force for the Fight Against Drug Trafficking, which would now control both military and police anti-drug forces, would be under police command. In 1990 one US official was so exasperated at the squabbling that he said he believed the Bolivian army was a major hindrance to anti-drug operations and that they would enjoy more success if it were completely excluded.[18] Also, the DEA has built up close relations with UMOPAR and put tremendous efforts into turning it into a corruption-free force. Forging similar links with the military could take years.

By the end of 1990, when the Bolivian government was still dithering, US officials were getting impatient. 'We cannot wait years and years for them to decide,' said one. By April 1991 they could wait no longer. By now a new factor had entered the equation: the Gulf War. The war had given Uncle Sam back the confidence in his political and military strength which had been so cruelly shattered by Vietnam. Having 'kicked Saddam's butt', it wasn't going to pussyfoot over how to tackle Bolivia's cocaine lords.

Less than a month after a cease-fire was reached between Iraq and the allied powers, President Paz Zamora announced that two army battalions (around 1,000 men in total) would enter Washington's other war, the war on drugs, after being trained by US military instructors. The move was rapidly pushed through Congress. In fact, the Congress debate was a bit of a formality as it turned out that the first 12 US military instructors, along with 180 tonnes of equipment and weapons, had already arrived the week before. Another 44 arrived a fortnight later. They were replaced by another team of around 59 advisors in October who trained 409 men in Riberalta. 'We are a small dependent country,' admitted one senior government official the day after the measure was approved. 'We don't have the power to resist US pressure.' The soul-searching was over. On 3 October the Bolivian army took part in its first drugs raid on the plains of the northern Beni.

6

Paying the Price:
The Addicts

Cochabamba

IN COCHABAMBA on a park bench in colonial Plaza Colón, a gang of ragged boys in bomber jackets idle away the hot Saturday evening. They wolf-whistle at the couples who stroll among the palm trees and hibiscus bushes, or scuffle with rival gangs.

Suddenly they tense up as they spot a middle-aged man in a suit. They watch him walk round the square a couple of times, but both parties are careful to avoid eye contact for the moment. Then the man gives a wink and one of the boys darts forward, pulling a tiny white packet out of his jacket. The man glances around nervously then presses a few crumpled notes into the boy's hand before disappearing up a dark alley. The deal has been sealed in seconds.

Later, a taxi-cab stops beside the square. One of the gang runs over, exchanges a few words and climbs in. The car slowly circles the square and the boy jumps out again to join his anxiously watching friends.

The boys belong to the growing army of children who live on the streets of Cochabamba, Bolivia's third largest city 110 miles southwest of the Chapare, consuming and selling *pitillos*, i.e. cigarettes of unrefined coca paste which are smoked pure or mixed with tobacco. The children, some as young as six years old, are paying the terrible price of Bolivia's cocaine boom.

Most begin by using cocaine, but once addicted are forced to turn to selling and stealing to finance their habit. On the streets, they work in a strict hierarchy. Only the top boys do the selling. The rest work as bodyguards, look-outs, or 'employees', which means they do whatever they are told. The guy with the most drugs and who is best at fighting becomes boss. Today the title is held by an 18-year-old addict nicknamed *El Gordo* (fatty). 'He's the top dog at the moment,' says one gang member, a boy called Carlitos. 'But if someone else turns up with more drugs, he'll become boss instead.'

Carlitos, an attractive 14-year-old with mischievous brown eyes and a sly sense of humour, began using and selling when he was eight after running away from home because his drunkard father and stepmother were squabbling. He joined a gang as an apprentice and gradually worked his way up. Today, he roams the streets night and day, endlessly in search of the magic white powder. He buys it at night, a kilo at a time, from a private house, then divides it into one-gramme piles which he wraps in paper torn out of school exercise books and packs into boxes of 12. He sells the one-gramme *sobres* for around ten *bolivianos* ($3), to anyone who wants them: policemen, businessmen, taxi drivers, other street boys. Recently, he says, paste prices have slumped because there is too much of the stuff around. He always keeps some back for himself. He reckons he gets through about 24 *sobres* a day.

Carlitos pays for his habit by stealing, or, in the local street slang, *lanzeando*. He began by breaking into houses, but has now been promoted within the gang to robbing old ladies of their jewellery in the street. At the end of the month he waits outside the offices of employees who have just picked up their pay cheques. But his favourite centre of operations is La Cancha, a street market where imported contraband goods are sold as a means of recycling drug dollars. In a section known as *Miamicito* (Little Miami), you can find anything from Christian Dior perfumes to Barbie dolls to Sony video recorders. Protected by a couple of look-outs, Carlitos filches the goods from the stalls and resells them a few days later. His other favourite trick is to trip up US tourists, then to empty their pockets as they recover from the shock.

He works with a guy called Pixchote, who has a reputation as the best *lanzero* in town. 'Pixchote can steal from the tightest pair of jeans,' says Carlitos. 'Everyone respects him, because he always has money. They know they can go to him when they need cash. He always helps them out.'

Some days, Carlitos is too stoned to do anything at all. Crouched on the rubbish-laden banks of the River Rocha, which runs through the centre of Cochabamba, he spends days just smoking from a pipe made from silver paper from the inside of cigarette packets. He goes days without food, then binges, stealing whole roast chickens from restaurants. He rarely sleeps. When he does, he just crashes out wherever he happens to be. Usually it is under the bushes in the Plaza Colón, or with the rats on the riverbanks. But unlike many of his friends, Carlitos takes care of himself. He dresses smartly and washes his hair every day; he knows it's better for business. He steals his clothes from La Cancha, or buys them with cocaine.

The *pitillo* trade is not restricted to boys. Many of the vendors and buyers are girls, who know their sex makes them less likely to be picked up by the police. They pay for their cocaine with their bodies.

Every few days the police round the children up, usually after middle-class inhabitants have complained that they are soiling the city's reputation. If the kids can afford it, they pay the police off; ten to fifteen *bolivianos* ($3 to $5) is the going rate. Sometimes the police pose as taxi drivers and lure the boys into deals. 'You have to be very careful,' says Carlitos. 'You learn to sell only to people you recognise.' Street children who can't pay are dragged off to a detention centre inside the central police station. Packed 40 to a cell with hardened criminals, the only food they get is what is brought by their families (if they have one) or by charity organisations like the Roman Catholic Amanecer, partly funded by the British government. The stench of urine is overpowering. 'They beat us with soup spoons to make us talk,' says one child, a 17-year-old called Rodolfo. 'A few days later they realise there's no point in holding us any more, so they let us go.'

No statistics exist, so no-one knows the true number of addicts in Cochabamba or in Bolivia as a whole. Estimates by the Cochabamba Municipal Council's Commission on Drug Addiction put the number in the city at between 3,000 and 5,000 (around 1 per cent of the population) with thousands more occasional users. Charity workers say they believe as many as 10 per cent of the population may be addicted, at least half of them children, with up to a third of the population occasional users. In Bolivia as a whole, the US embassy estimates that up to 10 per cent of Bolivia's population are occasional users and 3 per cent addicts.

Whatever the figures, addiction in Cochabamba and the Chapare is reaching alarming levels as increasing amounts of cheap paste swamp the market as a result of law enforcement and over-production. Often the children, like stompers in the Chapare, are victims of a deliberate strategy by traffickers to encourage addiction as a way of getting rid of their surplus. Sometimes the traffickers are policemen who resell their seizures. They prefer small-scale dealing through friends and contacts which lessens the chance of their being betrayed by rival traffickers. Ironically, law enforcement is making things worse: with the disruption of their normal routes, traffickers are unloading their cocaine onto the domestic market instead.

As much as 10 per cent of Bolivia's coca paste is diverted into domestic consumption, according to US sources. As addictive as 'crack', it is even more dangerous because it still contains a high proportion of impurities. 'Many of these kids are being poisoned not by the coca paste but by the horrific chemical impurities inside it, like ether, kerosene and even mercury,' says a US official.

According to Sister Stephany Murray, an American nun who runs Amanecer, which provides shelter for the street children and distributes milk and bread on the streets, addiction tends to be rooted in poverty and family problems. 'The kids leave home because there is nothing to eat or because they're being maltreated by their parents. They try to escape their reality. They start shining shoes, they lose contact with their families and they find it easier to steal or sell *pitillos*.' After that it is a downward spiral into a life of addiction, theft and squalor. Other addicts learn their habit while stomping coca leaves. Many are paid partly in paste.

It is not just the poor who become addicts. In the city's public high schools and universities the habit has spread like wildfire. 'It's very fashionable among the rich,' says Ana María Marañon, director of the Reto Juvenil rehabilitation centre. 'At parties they pass cocaine round in a large glass bowl. You'll find doctors, businessmen, even army generals who sniff it.'

Local and national authorities have done little to tackle the addiction problem, leaving it to religious charities and private individuals to cope. This is partly because they lack resources. Also, because coca paste is illegal, the government has left it to the police, rather than to health organisations, to treat and rehabilitate addicts. Another reason may be that politicians are reluctant to acknowledge the gravity of the problem. 'Bolivia's politicians don't accept the country has a problem, just as in the US we tried to deny we had one, until we had no choice,' says a US official. 'This may be one reason the Bolivian government is reluctant to be as tough in fighting drugs as we would like them to be.' Some Bolivians, on the other hand, say the US is exaggerating the addiction problem in order to counter Bolivia's argument that the root of the cocaine boom is US demand. Other Bolivians argue that although addiction is a tragic reality, it is a small problem compared to other problems facing Bolivia's impoverished people, like malnutrition, disease and unemployment.

For officials at the US embassy, convincing Bolivia it has an addiction problem is seen as the key to getting it to cooperate in fighting drugs. With this in mind, the embassy has set up a large number of public-awareness and drug-prevention campaigns, funded by agencies like USAID and the US Information Service. These include publicity spots and educational soap operas on Bolivian television, materials for schools and training courses for local leaders.

Until recently, the only centres where addicts were sent were run by the police or religious charities. 'Addicts had the choice between the stick or the Bible,' says a Santa Cruz journalist who has covered the subject. Those destined for the stick treatment are kidnapped and sent to camps misleadingly called *granjas de rehabilitación*, or rehabilitation centres. Run along the same lines as Soviet labour camps, the 'reformatories' were set up under an obscure law, passed in 1886, known as the Police Law, which allowed the Bolivian police to incarcerate anyone they considered anti-social. This covered drug addicts to vagrants to petty criminals, or anyone the police just did not like. They could be detained without trial for up to 12 months. In theory the police were forbidden to incarcerate children, but this was ignored. Often the children's parents themselves, unable to cope with their addiction and anti-social habits, pay police to abduct them.

The most notorious was called La Granja de Los Espejos (The Farm of Mirrors). Set up in 1967, it was run as a slave labour camp whose taskmasters could have walked straight out of Dickens. Surrounded by thick jungle and rivers, and virtually inaccessible by road, Los Espejos was cut off from the outside world.

One of its inmates was a British man named Philip Williams. He had spent a solitary life wandering the world, working as a trucker in Saudi Arabia and Pakistan, running a folk club in Amsterdam, ending up as a logger in the jungles of Bolivia. In 1989 he was working as a night watchman in a butcher's shop in Santa Cruz. One night, as he ambled from one of his favourite hangouts across the square at the start of his shift, a truck loaded with armed police pulled up in front of him and hauled him off. He lost consciousness. The next thing he knew he was in a police cell and was then driven 35 kilometres along a dirt jungle track to Los Espejos. There the guards forced him to work on a plantation whose name they had chosen in honour of their British guest: Las Malvinas.

An article on Williams in The *Independent Magazine*[1] described his life in the camp:

> At Granja de Espejos there were maybe 125 inmates. You had the criminal element in there, but you also had kids of 15 and 16. They called these the *palomillos* (the little doves).
>
> Answerable only to their immediate superiors, the camp guards, all of them low-ranking members of the police, were virtually a law unto themselves, free to indulge in random acts of sadism, and even murder. Their preferred weapon, according to Williams, was a thing called the 'gummy', a strap made of rubber taken from truck tyres. The guards plied the gummy entirely indiscriminately, it seemed to Williams.
>
> The prisoners spent their days raising livestock — pigs, sheep, chickens and ducks, clearing acres of the jungle around the camp and tending small vegetable patches. None of the prisoners profited from their labours. On the contrary, when the camps [later] came under public scrutiny... it was reported that most of the prisoners showed signs of severe malnutrition. Speculation was rife among the inmates as to where all the produce went.
>
> Without medical provision of any kind, undernourished and overworked, beaten on the smallest pretext, the internees led a demoralising and perilous life. As Williams explains: 'I was put in the "junkie" dormitory. There was always trouble in the junkie dormitory, half the people there should have been in special clinics. We started work at 6.00 a.m. and finished at 6.00 p.m. The food was pigswill. It was practically water. They threw in a couple of carrots and they would go to the slaughterhouse and come back with rotten cows' heads and throw them in 45-gallon drums, that was how they did the cooking there. If the sergeant was pissed off, at 4.30 a.m. they'd run you down to the river for bathing and the guards would have cut switches from eucalyptus saplings. They'd give you three to get into the river, and say really quickly "one, two, three", and of course you couldn't get even near to the river in that time, and they'd wade in and lash you with the saplings. From my time in the camp, I've got a fractured skull and ankle and there's something wrong with my ribs.'

Since 1984 reports had been filtering out of Los Espejos and other *granjas* of torture, unexplained deaths, and the imprisonment of children. From Los Espejos also came rumours of a secret burial site. Bolivian human rights groups alerted Amnesty International and a team of Argentine forensic anthropologists whose work following the 'Dirty War' at home had made them expert in exhuming tortured human remains.

Investigators concentrated their efforts on a small hill, 25 metres from the camp, topped with a cross. The inmates called it El Platanal, the Banana Grove. Climbing its steep sides, they found scores more crosses, some of wood, others of metal, and a patch of ground whose peculiar depressions and ridges (clearly man-made) aroused their suspicions. The scientists unearthed the complete remains of four people and the foot of a fifth, but estimated that in total El Platanal contained about 40 bodies. All bore signs of being beaten on the head or ribs with a blunt instrument. One had a bullet lodged in its skull.

While they were at the camp, the investigators noticed a solitary *gringo*. This was Williams, who, after nearly 11 months in captivity was in wretched shape and in urgent need of medical care. One day, he said, five guards had beaten him over the head with the butt of a rifle and kicked his teeth out simply because he was a *gringo*. Williams, now 51, had been powerless to contact the British embassy, which might have helped him get out. Escape was impossible.

> While I was there, several people tried to escape. They'd hide out in the bush during the day and then try to leg it when it got dark. The police would wait until night and then go out with lanterns and guns. They were allowed to shoot anyone trying to escape. It was highly dangerous to make for the road to Santa Cruz because the locals would report anyone for the sake of a few pesos. If you managed to get up through the forest in the other direction, you could, if you were lucky, make it to a colony of Dominican nuns, who knew about the camp and would help anyone get away from it. But they were a long way away.

Following the outcry over the cemetery, the Granja de Espejos was closed down in 1989. The inmates were loaded onto trucks, given five *bolivianos* each, and told to get out quick if they did not want trouble. The camp's governor, Lieutenant Colonel Luis Camacho, and five other policemen were charged with unlawful killing. Two lawyers who had helped in the closing, meanwhile, received death threats.

Of the four other *granjas*, one, La Granja de Chimoré, in the heart of the Chapare, is still open. It is run by a burly black police officer called Martín Gira, whom the inmates nickname Idi Amin or El Negro. Most of its detainees are youths who became addicted after stomping coca in towns like Villa Tunari and Sinahota. None has been formally charged. If they are not criminals when they enter, they certainly are when they leave.

When prisoners arrive they are 'baptised' with 30 lashings from a rubber whip bound with barbed wire. 'They do this so you will know what will happen to you if you escape,' says Manuel, an ex-inmate. Forced to get up at four, they are sent into the fields, often in temperatures of over 40 degrees, to cultivate crops or chop timber. They are paid nothing. 'They hit us as we worked,' recalls Manuel. 'It was like a race. If you finished last, you got extra beatings. Sometimes they used us for target practice. They would make us run and see if they could hit us.'

Inmates who disobey orders are punished with the 'pig' or the 'dry stick'. The 'pig' torture involves doing a press-up. If the prisoner moves or falls, he is beaten on the stomach. The 'dry stick' is even worse: the inmate has to stand in an ant-hill. 'When a prisoner is given the pig the guards warn the others "This is what will happen to you all if you tell on us or try to escape,"' says Manuel. In fact, those who try to run away face worse: many are shot dead. 'When people try to escape, the police say "Let's finish your coffin,"' says Manuel. 'I myself made two coffins. Of course, those who can afford it, pay to get out. The going rate is between $100 and $500.' In 1987 Amnesty investigated the death, presumably after trying to escape, of a 16-year-old inmate called Cleomedes Claros. His death certificate said he had died of 'acute anaemia' and 'severe bruising'. Other inmates said he had been beaten to death with a broom handle.

Others die of 'natural' causes, like tuberculosis or starvation. Food is disgusting. 'They fed the prisoners on chicken feed or yucca soup,' says Manuel. He admits he was lucky: he was given special food because he was dating the director's niece, Blanca. Sometimes he even ate meat. Although the inmates produced milk and vegetables by the tonne, they consumed none. 'The food we produced would have fed an entire city. Yet we were starving,' says Manuel. A delegation from Bolivia's Permanent Assembly for Human Rights described the prisoners they saw on a visit in 1990: 'Their physical appearance was ghastly. They had cuts on their hands and feet. One skinny lad had signs of advanced tuberculosis. Most were severely malnourished, and showed the signs of cumulative exhaustion after days of working in unbearable tropical heat.'

At night, according to Manuel, inmates sleep 30 or 40 to a cell. 'We were piled up one on top of the other like firewood.' Minors are regularly sexually abused. Manuel recounts how a man nicknamed Tripa Seca (Dry Tripe) would approach young boys and pull down their trousers. 'If they refused to have sex, he stabbed them.'

According to Manuel, police officers also ordered prisoners to process cocaine for them. 'They made us stomp coca. They would then market the cocaine. As policemen they had all the necessary contacts.' In 1986 the body of a 15-year-old inmate, whose death was investigated by Amnesty, was found to bear corrosive marks on his feet. 'The marks suggested... that he had been engaged in treading coca leaves to make paste,' said an Amnesty report. 'There were suspicions that he might have been deliberately killed to prevent him disclosing such activities.'

My name is Ricardo Arraya. I am 25 years old, from an ordinary middle-class cochabambina family. Seven years ago I had a promising career ahead of me as an industrial chemist and was just about to finish my university studies. Then one day I had toothache.

I had always been afraid of the dentist so I didn't want to go. Then a friend came up to me at college. 'If you take drugs, it will calm your gums,' he said. I tried marijuana and it worked. Then, whenever my gums hurt I looked for the guy. 'It'll do you good to smoke,' he said. I didn't know it, but he was a dealer. He knew he could get good money because my family was rich, so he wanted to make me an addict.

At first I just smoked when the tooth hurt. But soon it was every day. I began to stay at home, ignoring my friends who tried to get me back to college. I told my parents I was going to my room, and sat in there smoking. When my father realised what was happening, he said 'I'm not going to help you because you're a good-for-nothing.' I told him he had to support me until I was 21 because that was the law. So he did.

But soon the money ran out and I began to steal. One day I stole two crystal glasses from my family but I felt so bad afterwards I went out and replaced them. Instead I stole in the street, from cars, from passers-by, just to have enough money to get me through that day. I learnt how to open car doors with pieces of wire. It was exciting: when I stole I felt a thrill in my shoulders. It was almost more exciting than drugs. Sometimes the police caught me and my mother had to come and collect me. She would take me home and give me food. She got terribly upset.

One day I tried cocaine base. That was really the drug of all drugs. I couldn't leave it. All I could think about were those ten seconds of incredible pleasure. The rest was horrible suffering of my nerves. I forgot the values of people around me. I learned how to lie with the greatest of ease. I felt as if I would kill, just to alleviate the suffering I was going through. There was stacks of coke around, it was pouring into the city every single day, but the problem was getting it. I turned to alcohol to calm my nerves, becoming addicted twice over.

In the end, my family barred me from the house. I could go to my room but nowhere else. I had stopped eating and was getting very thin. I lost my friends. At the beginning we had smoked together, but now I just wanted to be alone. I wandered around the city with the stray dogs and slept in the hills. My clothes were in rags and I looked like a tramp: how I looked was the last thing I cared about. Gradually I realised I was in a prison: I wasn't happy anywhere. When it was day, the noise made me mad and I wanted the night. When it was night, the silence drove me to despair. I tried to break out. But even when I didn't try to buy drugs, people gave it to me. I couldn't say No.

When I was 22 I met Rosa at a party. Afterwards she came back to my room. She saw me smoking a pitillo, and asked what it was. 'Try it,' I said. So she did. A week later we got married. It seemed like the best way out. She had a good job as a clerk at the Central Bank. If I marry her, I thought, she'll look after me. We spent the honeymoon stoned on drugs and alcohol.

A few weeks later some friends from the Beni came to see me and told me about a 'nice little job' in the Chapare, earning easy money. So my wife left the bank and we moved to Eteramazama. I bought drugs *from the peasants then sold it to the* narcos *at a profit; they would ring to tell us when and where they were going to land their plane and we would load them up with drugs. For every seven kilos I bought, I'd make one in profit. But I never had any money because I used it all to buy drugs for myself.*

One day Rosa and I had a fight and she walked out. She was pregnant and went back to Cochabamba. I fell right down. By day I bought and sold drugs, at night I slept in the jungle. I caught yellow fever and my mother sent me a doctor from Santa Cruz. He managed to get me better but told me to stop smoking. Of course I couldn't.

I've always had an inclination for women. So I got myself a girlfriend, an attractive woman from Santa Cruz called Carmen. But the other men in the village where I worked got jealous. One night, one of them came to look for me in a room I was renting. 'Get that man out,' he told the owner, 'he's a good-for-nothing'. When the owner refused, the man got angry and stormed upstairs with a nine millimetre revolver in his hand. I was asleep. The man pointed the pistol at my head. 'You can't shoot a sleeping man,' the landlord pleaded. The man left sullenly. That saved my life. He'd certainly have killed me had I been awake.

A year or so later, Rosa came to visit me. She brought our child, a beautiful daughter, now one and a half years old. I decided to leave Carmen and go back to Cochabamba with Rosa. Soon we were back to our same old ways. I drank and took drugs to forget Carmen. I wanted to kill myself.

La Paz

Sunday is visiting day at San Pedro prison in La Paz. From 8.00 a.m. buxom Indian women in black bowlers and plaits jostle for position in front of the iron gates, rubbing their hands to fight off the early morning cold and taking it in turns to look through the peepholes. One woman with a big cloth bundle knocks. A pock-faced guard opens the gate a few inches and sticks his chin out. '¿Qué es?' (What is it?) he grunts. 'Can you pass this parcel in to my husband,' she asks. The guard slams the door in her face before she can finish her sentence. 'Visiting time is ten,' he growls from inside.

As the bells in the church across the Plaza San Pedro strike ten, the queue, now several hundred long, trickles in. Men and women enter through different sides to be searched for drugs or weapons. Often the guards find cocaine strapped to the women's inner skirts, or packed inside loaves of bread. On the other side of a second gate, prisoners watch anxiously to see if they have any visitors. Their faces look like a Goya painting: there are ghastly pale faces like skulls, scarred ones, broken despairing ones. All tell a secret tragedy.

Built to take 300 prisoners 100 years ago, San Pedro now houses over 1,300. Inside it is like a mini city, divided into six sections, each with its own exercise yard, restaurants, shops and set of cells. Like any ordinary city, money determines where you live. There are up-market areas with gardens and clean toilets like Los Pinos (The Pines) and La Posta, where the drug kingpins, like Roberto Suárez, live. For the middle-ranking prisoner there are sections like Alamos (Elms) and Guanay, which even have cinemas on Saturday nights. Last night's choice was between *Violación* (Rape) and *Las Chicas del Fuego* (Girls of Fire). Hard-core criminals go to the areas called San Martín and Palmar.

Those who can afford it buy themselves a cell (a good one costs $200) which they do up with wallpaper and any scraps of furniture they can find. They resell them at a profit when they leave. Prisoners like Suárez even have televisions and private kitchens, or eat in restaurants run by other prisoners. Poor ones sleep in the open pavilion with the rats and open sewers. They have no option but to eat the pale green slop the guards serve out of big iron cauldrons, which passes as lunch.

Around half of San Pedro's inmates are in for drug trafficking, although few of them are big fish of course. Most are stompers, paste carriers and the like who were too poor to pay off the police. But far from being reformed by San Pedro, most are utterly corrupted. For the prison is one of the most important cocaine trafficking and consumption centres in La Paz.

According to prisoners, cocaine is smuggled in by the police: usually stuff they have seized in raids and want to resell. 'They bring in most of the cocaine through the front door,' says one prisoner who calls himself Flaco (Skinny). 'If they don't want to bring it in themselves, they get women to take it in for them. Sometimes the police are caught and sent to prison. But that's only the few policemen the public find out about,' he adds.

Inside, the drugs are distributed by prisoners, usually experienced traffickers who make huge profits. 'You can tell them a mile off,' says Flaco. 'They're well-off compared to the misery of all the others. Often they run restaurants or shops to cover up their business.'

According to prisoners, cocaine is also processed in the prison. Precursors required for processing are brought in as medicines. 'There are an awful lot of sick people in here,' says Flaco sarcastically. Sometimes, he adds, prisoners cut cocaine base with insecticide to make it go further, with disastrous consequences for consumers. 'The traffickers are assassins.'

The dealers have a ready market. Most inmates see the white powder as the only way out of their squalor. Flaco reckons that between 60 and 80 per cent of inmates are addicted. Far from banning consumption, the prison guards, who do well out of it, encourage it. Cocaine is dirt cheap. A one-gramme *sobre* of coca paste, for example, costs between 50 and 70 *centavos* (20 US cents). For those in search of a superior high, a *sobre* of base costs around five *bolivianos* ($1.50).

Enslaved to cocaine, prisoners quickly degenerate. The worst ones congregate in a cell block called Siberia. 'They call it that because there is so much mist — in their heads,' jokes Flaco. 'They forget if it is day or night.'

To pay for their habit, inmates rob their fellow prisoners. Or they go to money lenders (usually the same dealers) who charge extortionate rates of interest. 'Once a prisoner starts borrowing, he's ruined,' says Flaco.

> They lend you ten *bolivianos*. The next day you have to pay back 20, the next day 40. The worst thing is that when a prisoner asks for a large amount of credit, he has to promise to consume a corresponding amount of drugs every day. If he doesn't, the bastards start charging him interest on the spot regardless of whether he can pay. Some have to pay with their bodies, they allow the dealer to rape them in exchange for being let off a debt.

After that it's a steady downward spiral, as one former prisoner addict, called Antonio, found to his cost. He became so hardened by his addiction, he no longer cared about anything. 'All I wanted was to get stoned. I didn't care if I hurt someone or killed him. I'd become really vicious. I no longer cared about anything, whether I was in for a long time or a short time. Life meant nothing.' He saw several prisoners die. 'Prisoners killed each other for the slightest thing,' he says. 'They used knives or gave people dope which had been poisoned. The bodies were thrown over the balconies. If the man had any family, they came to collect the body. Otherwise they just went straight to the cemetery.'

Antonio realised that if he stayed any longer in San Pedro he would not get out alive. On the other hand, though, he was frightened of the idea of being outside where he would not be allowed to get stoned all day long.

> It was a mixed feeling. During the day, I preferred being in the prison because I knew I could consume without being bothered. But after six when they locked the doors and it got dark, I was afraid for my life. That was when the Mafia who worked for the traffickers started demanding money and killed people who hadn't paid up.

Antonio was fortunate. His sentence expired and he was sent to a rehabilitation centre in the Chapare. Most others in San Pedro are not so lucky.

7

The Thrill Seekers:
The DEA

Trinidad

BOB Johnstone takes a packet of popcorn out of the microwave oven, its contents transformed from tiny yellow seeds to puffy white snowflakes. The popcorn, flown in specially from the US, is one of the few consolations in this Wild West jungle town. As chief DEA agent in the Beni city of Trinidad, in the heart of cocaine country, Bob needs a few treats to keep him going. It is 9.00 in the morning but Bob has already done two-and-a-half hours' work, planning which of the area's huge cocaine labs to target and trying to communicate with the embassy in La Paz over a radio connection so scratchy the voices sound as if they come from Mars.

He disappears without a word into the tiny radio room next door. Bob has little time to chat with his team of Snowcap agents in T-shirts and running shorts slumped in comfy chairs around the room. Anyway, they are fully absorbed by a video: *Life and Death in LA*. Today they are lucky; it is a new one. One of the agents brought it from Texas when he was posted here three weeks ago. Lost into a fantasy world of Californian gangster warfare, ironically only a little different from what they do in real life, the agents are oblivious to the crackle of the radio and the drone of the motor-bikes in the steamy streets outside.

The Snowcappers have turned the room into a little bit of the US. The shelves are crammed with Tom Clancy novels. The agents are particularly tickled by his latest, *Clear and Present Danger*, which takes the war on drugs as its theme. 'It's actually quite accurate,' says one agent. Beside the novels are neatly stacked bottles of ketchup and Tabasco sauce, tins of tuna and packets of Marlboro cigarettes, all imported. Then there are trophies of war. On the far wall is a bull's skull picked up during a Beni raid. From one horn hangs a plastic chicken, from the other a propeller. 'Death From Above: DEA Air Wing', reads the caption. Then there's the 'fun barometer', a homemade contraption on which agents register their thrills with a cardboard pointer. At the bottom of the scale is 'Oscar Brain Dead'. It graduates through 'boring' and 'normal' to 'much fun' and 'danger', and finally 'Kenny Roy'. Someone has scrawled on it, 'Warning, fun light is on!'

There is a knock at the door. Jaime,[1] an Hispanic American from Miami who does most of the Spanish-speaking for the group, drags himself away from the latest shootout. *'Pasa'* (come in), he mutters. A humourless young woman in a white apron enters and silently puts a tray onto the table. On it are pots of coffee, fruit salads and piles of white toast, served with mock silver cutlery and starched white linen napkins. The woman thrusts a handful of bills onto the table. Without removing their eyes from the video, the agents push wads of *boliviano* notes into her hand without bothering to count them.

It is breakfast time in the Hotel Ganadero, a white Florida-style building on Trinidad's main street. The hotel, whose name means the Ranchers' Hotel, is the smartest in town. Apart from cocaine, ranching is Trinidad's biggest business. No-one quite knows if the hotel was built with ranching or cocaine money, but then people here rarely bother to ask. The more facetious DEA agents who claim to know of the hotel's other activities call it the Hotel Gonorrhea.

For the hotel's managers the DEA is good business, though they admit the gun-toting Americans may scare off some customers. Johnstone pays them $15,000 a month for the two floors, but says the hotel is always raising the price. 'They keep trying to put up the rent, while the service gets worse and worse,' he complains. 'Each time we threaten to leave. Once we actually did. We moved back a few months later.'

As a DEA temporary base, the Ganadero is several cuts above the prefabs of Chimoré. Occupying two entire floors,[2] the agents live a life of air-conditioned luxury only dreamed of by their colleagues in the Chapare. The day room, the farthest room on the third floor, is a converted bedroom, the radio room once a bathroom. The bedroom next door is now an office where sensitive communications equipment and computers are kept. Bob Johnstone sleeps there too. 'Entry only to authorised DEA personnel and their guests,' warns a notice on the door. The other rooms are agents' bedrooms. Pairs of huge black army boots are parked outside their doors for the shoeshine boy who comes by three times a week.

Although Snowcappers try to keep a low profile, every druglord knows that the Hotel Ganadero, like the Plaza hotel in La Paz and the Marriott in Panama City, is the 'DEA hotel'. In case a trafficker should decide to pay a visit, each floor is sealed off with solid iron gates which are locked at night. Dozy Leopards keep a 24-hour guard in the corridor while watching dubbed American films on television.

BACK IN the day room, the video has finished and the day's work is beginning. Six agents change their running shorts and Reeboks for combat fatigues and big black boots. They are to raid a laboratory about an hour and a half by helicopter north of Trinidad which an informant has said belongs to the Roca family. Two agents camouflage their faces with black war-paint and tie kerchiefs round their foreheads like characters out of a cowboy movie. 'The paint's not strictly necessary,' admits the team leader, a brawny Hispanic called Rich. 'But it makes them feel like Rambos. These guys are fed up they didn't get to fight in the Gulf War. They want to make up for it now.'

If they flew to the lab, the *narcos* and their workers would hear the chopper engines and be long gone by the time the agents arrived. Instead, they will be dropped in the jungle and will 'infiltrate'; they will spend two or three days creeping through thick forest in search of a clandestine airstrip or lab. Three days is usually the limit because carrying food and water for more makes too much clatter.

'Are the UMOPARs ready?' Bob Johnstone asks Rich. 'How many are coming?'

'Yeah, they're meeting us at the airport. There's eight of them. They're bringing a *fiscal* [prosecutor] too.'

'Holy shit,' says Bob. 'I told the *comandante* there wasn't room for him. He always insists that guy comes.'

One agent, a blond-haired Texan called Rob, wolfs down a vast plate of beef stew and noodles. 'My last proper meal for several days,' he says mournfully. 'From now on it's MREs [Meals Ready to Eat].' He turns to the Rambo who is assembling boxes of MREs and drinking water. 'By the way, did you put in the turkey and ham loaf? It's my favourite. I'm sick of lamb curry. And don't forget to bring lots of chocolate.'

In the wilderness of the Beni, conditions will be tough. They may have to march through head-high elephant grass, their 40-pound packs on their backs, or stagger up to their chests through alligator-infested rivers in the dark trying to keep their guns dry. Their feet rot or are burrowed by hook worms, their bodies are riddled with mosquitoes and other insects. There are even moths that give them blisters as big as grapefruits. With luck they may find clandestine airstrips carved out of the trees, which they blow up with dynamite, sending clouds of brown earth hundreds of feet into the air. They may stumble across labs, hidden deep beneath the jungle canopy, and come home with their clothes and hair stinking of the chemicals. Or cocaine stashes, set up by the 'bad guys' as an insurance policy in case their labs get raided. Often, though, the agents find nothing, because their intelligence was wrong or because the traffickers' was better.

When they find labs, it can be hairy. Sometimes agents find 40 to 100 workers pointing automatic weapons at them. In September 1990 four DEA agents were caught in a two-and-a-half hour shootout with a gang of armed druglords in the Chapare and an agent was seriously wounded. Normally, though, the traffickers appear wary of taking on the well-trained *gringos*. 'They're scared to death of us. They know that if they shoot we would send the whole camp out,' says one. 'You look at them and they bawl.'

It is 11.00 a.m. and time to leave. The agents sling their packs onto their backs, grab their M-16s and water canteens and slip into the bustling street below. They load into Toyota trucks and make for the airport where they pick up the Leopards and fly off. For those left behind there is plenty to do. Like follow-up from a raid the night before. One agent updates seizure figures on a blackboard: base labs — 15, hydrochloride labs — 12, cocaine paste — 34 kilos.... Another sifts through photographs and videos of the raid and writes up reports which will be sent to the embassy in La Paz.

One agent prepares to meet an informant whom he is keen to cultivate. He takes a bottle of Coke with him in the hope it will make the guy more cooperative. Other agents crash into bed or relax by the pool, recuperating from a string of nights in the jungle. They swap stories and compare insect bite tallies. 'Did you see us?' asks one. 'We got lost. We never found the lab we were looking for. The goddam informant gave us the wrong info. I'm not using him again.'

'Those mosquitoes were something wicked,' adds another. 'You should see John's ankle, it's covered. He could be on the way to beating the record, 120 on one ankle.'

Bob Johnstone, meanwhile, is in the radio room planning the next day's operation with another Snowcapper to a background of ghoulish radio messages from the departing agents. Through the window Johnstone watches their two helicopters fly off into the jungle.

'How many helos [helicopters] will we have tomorrow?' asks the agent, a man called Ray from Arizona.

'Just the two. Number three is still out of action. They promised us the spare parts from Panama would get here today, but they still haven't arrived,' replies Bob.

'How many LBGs do we need?'

LBG, short for Little Brown Guys, is the term agents use to describe the Leopards. In contrast to Chimoré, Snowcappers in Trinidad have little contact with the Leopards, whose base is a couple of miles outside town. Even when they do venture into Trinidad, few Bolivians can afford the *gringo* hangouts, such as the *whiskería* in the Ganadero.

Ray admits that DEA agents are a rare breed. Independent as wildcats, they like their own company but also need excitement to keep them going. 'Much of the work is monotonous and boring but it's studded with a few moments of sheer terror when the adrenalin really flows,' he says. Most find it difficult to adapt to normal lives afterwards. 'You get used to living on the edge. Psychologists call us "thrill seekers,"' he says.

But it's definitely a young man's life. And agents quickly get burned out. 'Sometimes you're out in the jungle being eaten alive and it's pissing down with rain again, and you ask yourself "What the hell am I doing here?" Often I think I've had enough of playing cops and dopers and I ought to grow up. But the bug doesn't let you go.' In career terms, Bolivia is good too: a posting in the Andes is a sign that the boss believes in you, and usually leads to rapid promotion.

LOCATED in the heart of the Beni, and inaccessible by road, Trinidad is one of the remotest cities on earth. The only way to get here is by air. The four weekly flights from La Paz are fixed in the minds of the town's 50,000-odd inhabitants. Watching the plane skim the spires of the cathedral and the terracotta-roofed houses, they look forward to fresh stocks of beer and a change of conversation. They chuckle as they watch the new arrivals shed their fur coats, designed for the chill of La Paz, and adapt to the 40-degree heat.

Few tourists come here, and if they do they stay only a few days. As the guidebook warns, there's little to do and Trinidad is only worth visiting if you're in search of 'adventure and a change of pace'. Given Trinidad's reputation as a cocaine centre, there are some adventures that might be best avoided. The intrepid tourists brave the mosquitoes for a boat trip up the Beni's main river, the Mamoré, to the Chapare, hoping to spot the jaguars and pumas which live in the forests. Most prefer to hang around the seedy bars, listening to local gossip. But change of pace there is: apart from UMOPAR jeeps and the odd horse and cart, the only mode of transport is the motorcycle. At midday, when the heat intensifies, the city slumbers, interrupted only by the occasional drone of a small plane flying overhead (ranchers or drug traffickers, nobody knows which).

In 1986 Trinidad celebrated the 300th anniversary of its founding by Spanish missionaries. But the mayor is still trying to fathom out why they chose this site. When the rainy season begins around Christmas, the open sewers bordering the streets turn into impassable rivers of mud, which fill with croaking frogs and mosquitoes. Only the earth dyke which has been built around the town keeps it from disappearing completely under the flood waters.

The town revolves around the central square, a few blocks from the Ganadero. It is dominated by a fine colonial cathedral built by Spanish Jesuits in 1686. In the centre, old women in black shelter from the sun under the palm trees. Ice-cream sellers in white coats push their little carts, honking a horn to attract customers. Meanwhile, local youngsters ride their motorbikes round and round the square, dodging the pot-holes as they eye one another up. When it gets too hot, they drink coffee under the colonial arcades and watch the rest of the world go by.

Then there is the market, where pawpaws and pineapples are stacked beside imported jeans and T-shirts. Housewives come here to buy food for the cocaine labs in return for a little pocket money. Some prepare it too, handing it to respectable-looking middlemen who take it to the labs by river or small plane. Other locals supply chemicals, generators and other mechanical equipment.

Few of the profits from the drug trade, though, have filtered into the town. Trinidad is what Santa Cruz was like 20 years ago. There are no BMW dealerships or video rental businesses and only a handful of large houses. Trinidad is simply where the traffickers do business. They live and spend their money in Santa Cruz or Cochabamba.

Cocaine also has to compete with the city's other industry, ranching. Since the Jesuits brought cattle to Trinidad in the late 15th century, the city has been the centre of Bolivia's beef industry. The cattle thrived on the Beni's fertile grasslands which today nurture around three million head of cattle. Trinidad's Federation of Ranchers, with 5,000 members, became the town's main social centre. The ranchers fly the meat to La Paz and mining towns in the Andes in vintage Second World War planes. The pilots, who navigate the mountains often without radar, are among the best in the world.

In the early 1980s, when cocaine prices boomed, the ranchers came under pressure from the traffickers. Some had their ranches taken over at gunpoint and were forced to flee. Others joined the barons, using their cattle as a useful decoy. When the DEA arrived in the late 1980s, the druglords simply moved up-river to Santa Ana. 'Obviously the bad guys were annoyed when we went there,' says Johnstone. 'But the ranchers were pleased because we protected them. One had had his 45,000-hectare estate taken over.'

From the agents' point of view, Trinidad is a placid enough place, at least by day, and its inhabitants are an easy-going bunch. Unlike the highlanders, known as *collas*, the swarthy people of the Beni lowlands, known as *cambas*, are a fun-loving people who let *mañana* take care of itself.

In the early mornings, while it is still cool, the Snowcappers go jogging along the circular road or do weights. On idle days, they go up to the hotel pool or visit one of the local restaurants for beef steaks so large they spill off the plates. There's the Country Club too, just outside town beside a lagoon. You can swim there provided you avoid the crocodiles and brave the mosquitoes. Overall, though, there is so little to do that agents end up making lots of money. 'We get paid a *per diem* of $37, plus overtime. That's big bucks here,' says an agent. 'Over a three month assignment I reckon to save around $6,000.'

The locals view the Americans with the mixture of admiration and resentment with which people view any occupying force. For many, the agents are a source of income and, with luck, a US passport. Local women make a few extra dollars by giving them Spanish lessons (and other services). In Chimoré, mothers even name their babies after Snowcappers or their home towns. There's a Carolina Norte, even a Johnny Walker. 'They like us being here,' says Herschel, a Navy Seal.

> Some have lived in the US but came back. When I leave I give the guys I like my kit. They need it, I want them to survive. But I don't like them asking for it. This is their country and they'll never be Americans however much they try to imitate us. Sometimes they say 'Hey you earn so much *per diem*.' I tell them I couldn't even pay my electricity bill with what they earn. 'I'm lucky enough to come from the US. You are from Bolivia'.

Many local residents disagree. One claims the townspeople loathe the agents. 'They treat us "natives" like dirt and bring us prostitution,' he says. 'They don't report to anybody, think they own the place.' Some even buy the conspiracy theory that the agents are in fact drug traffickers. 'Why do they never attack the really big targets? Because they don't want to,' one says. Local journalists resent the fact that the DEA never takes them on raids. The only ones who are taken are hard-bitten US hacks who fly in for a day or two from Washington or Miami and are used by the DEA guys to impress their bosses back home. In fact, recently, they have been reluctant to take even them, preferring to keep the nitty gritty of DEA operations a secret.

The local army general, who is clearly concerned about the growing strength of the DEA and UMOPAR, is unhappy too. Once he tried to ban the agents from carrying guns in Trinidad. 'We spoke to the embassy, which explained to him that we all had licences,' says a Snowcapper. 'He eventually backed down and said he just wanted to be notified of our movements so that when locals complained about the helicopter noise he could explain. He must be kidding. We're not telling him a goddam thing.'

In the evenings, when the day-time heat subsides, Trinidad pulsates to the Afro-Caribbean rhythms of the Oriente (the eastern lowlands). The Snowcappers visit The Black Hole, a pub across from the Ganadero which reportedly doubles up as a brothel when necessary. 'The girls go wild, particularly when they see the Americans flash wads of greenbacks,' says a Trinidad resident. There are other fleshpots, but you need a good stomach to visit them. The seediest is La Peña Grande, a tumbledown shack in the unlit outskirts of town where miniskirted girls, many no older than 16, giggle nervously when they spot the *gringos*. For the choosier, but not too choosy, there is Los Duendes (The Gnomes), which poses as a night club and reeks of damp sheets.

Usually, the agents prefer the security of the hotel. They drink Paceña beers on the roof terrace overlooking the lights of the city, and beyond, the black expanse of the jungle. Or they gravitate to the *whiskería* where cocktails are better and attractive women in plentiful supply. Only the cream of Trinidad's females come here, most in search of husbands. 'Many of them see us as the key to a successful future, so they try to get hitched with one of us,' says one DEA agent. 'It's not uncommon for them to mention marriage as early as the second date. Sometimes even the first.'

Every few weeks, the agents leave the city for four or five days of Rest and Recuperation. Usually they go to Cochabamba, where there are plenty of luxury hotels with pools. Sometimes they go to Santa Cruz, but many find there are too many traffickers there to feel comfortable. 'You never know who is being paid to protect whom. You might come out of a bar and someone picks a fight, and you go to prison. It can take days to get out,' says an agent.

BOB JOHNSTONE, a soft-spoken Texan, does not look like a typical drug warrior. Six feet tall and in his early 40s, he wears pastel-coloured sweat shirts and is a dab hand at golf and moose hunting. Before taking over as temporary head of DEA operations in Trinidad, he was DEA boss in Santa Cruz for three and a half years. Before that he worked in the DEA's office for international training in Georgia.

When required, he can affect a sociable air. He knows how to give a good talk to US congressmen who pay lightning visits from Washington to check how their drugs war is going. He has a skilful hand too with the local military and police chiefs, never rising to the bait when their frustrations explode into bursts of rabid anti-Americanism. With informants, he has a knack for getting them to go places he would never dare to tread.

By nature, though, Johnstone is a loner, an attitude strangers mistake for rudeness. He is happiest locked up in the radio room keeping tabs on his agents in the jungle and discussing the next operations with his boss, Don Ferrarone, the DEA country attaché in La Paz.

For Johnstone, fighting the cocaine barons has become a way of life. He works from 6.00 or 7.00 a.m. until 11.00 p.m. seven days a week but never seems to get ahead. As soon as he gets through one case, another lands on his desk. Every day informants creep into the Ganadero to tell him of new labs that have sprung up like mushrooms. He rarely gets a chance to see his wife who lives in La Paz.

Despite the workload, Johnstone likes Trinidad's sleepy pace. In fact he says he would find it virtually impossible to get used again to the frenetic rush of US cities. A desk job at headquarters in Washington is his vision of hell on earth. After a month's annual leave, he is always relieved to be back doing what he most enjoys: busting dopers.

When Johnstone arrived in Bolivia in 1987, it was Colombia that was making headlines with spectacular seizures and shootouts between druglords and police. Few Americans realised that, meanwhile, Bolivia's cocaine Mafia was quietly growing in strength. The Bolivians, who had previously restricted themselves to exporting crude coca paste to Colombia for further refining, were now doing the processing themselves. From the day he arrived Johnstone realised Bolivia's growing importance as a major cocaine producer. But his facilities were terribly limited. He had no computer into which he could file the information passed onto him from informants. Instead he had to scribble it into notebooks and pass it on to the embassy by radio knowing it was being intercepted. 'Anyone who wanted to listen to my conversations only had to drop in to the radio station across the road,' he says. And the area he covered was huge; the departments of Beni, Pando and Santa Cruz combined were roughly the size of Texas. Slowly, things improved. Soon Johnstone had compiled a list of Bolivia's top traffickers.

When he arrived the cocaine king was still Roberto Suárez. He had the contacts with Colombia's Medellín cartel, so most of the smaller traffickers had to work through him. Then new names began to appear. There was Techo de Paja, Suárez's nephew, who stole most of Suárez's business, but in 1989 he disappeared. Other druglords turned up whom people back home had never heard of, like 'Lieutenant' Guzmán, 'Captain' Flores and Hugo Rivero.

New names popped up all the time. There were hundreds. Some were 'sleepers', traffickers who disappeared or laid low for a while then suddenly appeared again. Johnstone knew it was impossible to pursue all of them: he did not have the manpower. Whereas in the US he would have had ten men on a single case, here each agent had 20 traffickers from which to choose. Usually it was a matter of targeting the ones who popped up most often.

In 1987 the US decided to hit back and set up an operation codenamed Snowcap. It aimed to cut the amount of cocaine entering the US from the three Andean countries where most cocaine was grown and made (Bolivia, Peru and Colombia) by half over three years. DEA agents were sent for three months at a time, apart from a handful like Johnstone who stayed three or four years.

At first, the agents focused on destroying coca fields and 'mom and pop' cocaine paste labs in the Chapare. But soon they realised it would be more effective to target large labs, most of which were in the Beni. In theory if these labs were destroyed, *campesinos* would have no market for their leaves, prices would fall and they would turn to other crops. Politically, too, it was more acceptable to hit rich traffickers than dirt-poor *campesinos* who depended on coca for a livelihood. Agents gathered intelligence on trafficking networks and traced their assets in Bolivia and in the US. Snowcap helped change legislation too. It pushed through laws on precursor chemicals, for example, which entitled the US authorities to inspect the books of any US chemicals exporter.

From 1988 Johnstone was able to make use of other US agencies with expertise in areas like river and border patrols. Members of the US Border Patrol's special operations unit, Bortac, were sent to the Chapare to help search vehicles for cocaine and precursors. The US Coast Guard and Navy Seals and Seabees were brought into the Beni to train the Bolivian navy and UMOPAR commando units to carry out raids along the region's vast river network. A US army Special Forces Mobile Training Team provided training at Chimoré. Another group set up Operation Screaming Eagle, which identified and intercepted aircraft. US army Special Forces personnel were brought in as medics, engineers, mechanics and computer experts.

The biggest asset the military could offer was its expertise in intelligence gathering and the equipment and funds to do it. It provided Johnstone with the latest gadgets, like the Command and Management system which, using a computer programme codenamed Hawkeye, allowed field agents to photograph drug runners' planes with a digitalised camera, send the image through the computer system to Washington and learn the likely route and destination of the plane within minutes. Johnstone acquired computers into which he could key details of traffickers, drug operations and informants' tip-offs. He could even speak on the telephone with the embassy or the Pentagon without being intercepted. Radio messages were scrambled so that traffickers could not listen in. The military also promised to provide huge portable radar units which would be used to seal off the Chapare. Other equipment was so sensitive that the DEA refused to tell the media what it was.

The information DEA agents gleaned in the field was transmitted to a team of military intelligence analysts in the embassy in La Paz. 'The problem was that the DEA was generating intelligence but did not have the expertise to put it together. The military people were able to impose order on it,' says a US official. Recently the team, made up of combined Department of Defense and DEA personnel, was doubled in size from 12 to 24. They work in a huge operations room, its walls covered with charts of the Bolivian jungles. Using intelligence from the field and from Southern Command in Panama and the Pentagon, the analysts plan busts and plot them on the map with black dots, which are pitifully small against the vastness of the jungle. Sometimes they share some intelligence with a chosen few Bolivians.

Since Colombia tightened the screws on its traffickers in 1990, DEA officials claim some fled to Bolivia, bringing their violent methods and arms with them. Johnstone worries this could mean greater risks for his men. In the Chapare, agents always carry M-16s and pistols and move in pairs. But in Trinidad it is far more relaxed. 'The boys wander around town, go to restaurants, whore houses, wherever. Usually they go unarmed, or just carry a pistol,' Johnstone says. 'Nothing has happened to any of them yet but we've been lucky. That makes us assume that it's safe here and that nothing will happen. But that's not rational. We're likely to become targets soon. Someone will get shot.'

Johnstone never goes out without a gun. He has had his share of close shaves. One evening in 1989, a car drew up outside his house in Avenida Banzer in Santa Cruz. Robbie Suárez got out and walked to the door with a pistol. He shot at the guard at the door and shouted, 'You are protecting worse people than me,' then ran off. The next day local newspapers published details of the shooting, including the name and address of Johnstone whom they described as 'the most prominent agent in Bolivia'.

The next day Johnstone had a visit from his landlady who happened to be Carmiña Ortiz, Robbie's girlfriend. She tore up the lease and told him angrily he had three days to get out. That evening Robbie was shot dead by Bolivian police, but fingers automatically pointed at Johnstone, and Roberto Suárez put a $1 million contract on his life. All DEA agents are used to such threats, but Johnstone knew this one was serious. He was put on the first plane to Caracas, Venezuela, where he stayed for 30 days.

Stories like Johnstone's created paranoia at the embassy. All DEA officials and agency heads now carry guns and bodyguards which have become status symbols, like owning a Porsche. 'Gun fever appears to have taken over,' says an embassy official. 'It's a Rambo thing. Every one has to have one, even people who never go into the field.' Robert Gelbard, the US ambassador,[3] takes six bodyguards wherever he goes, even to football matches. His children live cooped up at home like caged lion cubs. All DEA agents based in La Paz have Bolivian police guards outside their homes, except one, Gene Castillo, the DEA's deputy country attaché. Castillo, an amiable man who keeps a can of 'bullshit repellant' next to his DEA medals, believes bodyguards are more of a liability than a protection. 'It's crazy,' he says. 'It just draws attention. A guy walks past your house and sees a guard outside. He says "Hey, that person must be important or rich. Let's go and see." He might try to kidnap your kids for a ransom.'

Johnstone is willing to run the risks because he believes the fight against the cocaine barons in Bolivia is a crucial part of the overall US war on drugs in the Andes. 'In Colombia the *narcos* have been in control for a long time,' he says. 'It's almost too late to do anything there. In Peru, the bad guys have won too. The crucial thing is to stop them taking over in Bolivia.'

It's a costly gamble: a single helicopter sortie costs over $1,000 and the Bolivian operation as a whole costs US tax-payers millions. But Johnstone believes he and his agents are beginning to make the traffickers hurt. 'We're making life difficult for them. Some are selling up in order to pay their debts to the cartels. They never know where we are going to strike next.'

His most important weapon is the intelligence he gets from informants. No-one likes or trusts a person who makes a living by betraying his or her friends but Johnstone knows DEA operations depend on them. He pays generously to make sure they come back. He believes in the saying 'Money talks, bullshit walks.' Informants come in all shapes and sizes. 'We have doctors, lawyers, bank clerks, *campesinos*. Some come to us because they need the money to survive or because they've got a grudge against a trafficker employer who has given them a bum deal.' Many are traffickers themselves.

Their stories lead Johnstone to cocaine laboratories or landing strips in the Beni jungle. Because of the wildness of the area, they are often difficult to track down. 'An informant will say "the lab is so-many hours' walk north east of such and such a town" but often that's not nearly specific enough for us to find it,' says Johnstone. Sometimes they just lie.

Following leads, Johnstone often stumbles across the tracks of Bolivian police and military units which are supposed to be cooperating with him. He plans a raid then finds the traffickers have been tipped off by a UMOPAR officer. In general, the police cooperate on the small cases. But when it comes to the big names, they become paralysed. 'Corruption permeates all levels of the anti-narcotics forces,' says Johnstone. 'A UMOPAR officer simply has to instruct his guys not to search some traffickers at a particular checkpoint for three days and he earns a lifetime's salary. Meanwhile they go out on ops with us in other areas to look as if they're doing something.' The navy and the air force are even worse. The frustrating thing is that the US can do very little about it.

But corruption is diminishing, say the agents, partly as a result of police officers being trained at the School of the Americas in Panama. 'We've come a long way in the past two years,' says one. 'Before, they would arrive at a lab, pick up the money and make a U-turn. Now they really want to get the dope and bust the bad guys.'

The other reason for the improvement is the US ambassador, Bob Gelbard. Unlike most diplomats, Gelbard is not afraid to say what he thinks, and that includes exposing crooked policemen whenever he hears about them. When he has to choose between drugs and diplomacy, drugs always win. Several times Gelbard has threatened to suspend US aid unless the government removes corrupt officers, effectively exercising a veto on all appointments. As a result, Johnstone is reasonably confident that the UMOPAR commanders in the Chapare and the Beni are clean. 'If I had to put my life on the line, I'd do it with them,' he says. He discusses plans for some operations with them. He shares morsels of intelligence, though never more than is necessary. Often the *comandantes* have to rely on their own intelligence, coordinated separately in La Paz.

Officially, the DEA is simply 'advising' the Bolivian anti-drugs forces on how to combat drugs by coordinating intelligence information. In their dealings with the Bolivian media, officials at the US embassy are instructed to 'stress that the DEA role is to support and assist the Bolivian police'.[4] In fact, although they have no powers of arrest or interrogation, the DEA has been on the front line ever since Snowcap began. No-one is in any doubt that it is the DEA, not UMOPAR, which pulls the strings, and to the resentment of senior police officers. 'Officially we are here as advisers,' says Johnstone. 'But everyone knows that is b—s—. We go out on all the important busts.'

Sometimes they overstep the mark, as in June 1991 when 20 DEA agents and 640 Bolivian police wrested Santa Ana from the control of the traffickers. The bust, codenamed Operation Safe Haven, was fairly successful (though no big traffickers were caught) but a couple of alleged actions by the DEA agents nearly got them booted out of Bolivia. In one, a DEA official was accused of taking part in an incident in which a Bolivian navy lieutenant was kicked, bound and gagged and left beside the road. In a second, a DEA agent supposedly broke into an army plane to test it for traces of cocaine. For many Bolivians, the raid and the alleged incidents demonstrated that the DEA, not the government of the country, was running the show. 'The special force for the fight against drug trafficking serves only US interests,' declared the Catholic radio station Fides the day after the raid. 'UMOPAR is not at the service of Bolivia, it is at the service of the US. Our government should put the DEA in its place. We need it, on this we are clear, but we do not need it to order us around, while we simply obey it.'

In the long term, DEA officials say their aim is to withdraw from involvement in paramilitary raids as soon as the Bolivian anti-drugs forces are adequately trained. The agents' role would become increasingly advisory. 'Unlike in El Salvador and Vietnam where we ran the show for them,' says one DEA agent in La Paz, 'in Bolivia we're trying to train them up so they can do things by themselves.' But officials admit that time is a long way off. Some, like Gene Castillo, fear it may never come. 'As long as we're involved as a hands-on presence, we can keep corruption down and people in gaol. If we go it's over.' Even if Bolivia did carry on the anti-drug war, it would be unlikely to conduct it in the way Washington wanted. The most likely scenario is that the DEA will pull out when the US has lost its obsession with cocaine.

RICHARD trains his eyes over the olive-green expanse of grassland 1,000 feet below. Ostrich-like birds, called ebus, scuttle into the undergrowth beside a wide river. On the far bank, Richard spots a row of huts, a half-built church and a jetty leading to a large boat. A stretch of green velvet beside the hamlet looks as if it could be the airstrip.

He manoeuvres the Casa transport plane to circle the town. Richard is one of the DEA's most experienced pilots. He served in Danang in Vietnam. The other qualifications listed on his 'alternative' visiting card include 'part time lover', 'all round good guy', 'casual hero' and 'singer of songs and ballads'. Today, though, his mind is on the simpler business of dropping off coast-guard agents to their mother ship on the river below.

'That should be Bella Vista if we're lucky. Can you see any red flares?' he asks Jim, the co-pilot.

'Nope,' replies Jim. Richard radioes the control tower in Trinidad, 40 minutes back. 'We're approaching a strip about 100 metres long, a quarter of a mile east of the town.' In the back, five Americans sprawled on the floor in their fatigues among the boxes of pasta and vegetables wake from their doze.

Suddenly a ball of pink fire explodes on the edge of the strip. 'That's it. OK, stand by,' says Richard. 'Just for the record let's fly over it once. Check for holes and any horses. Looks a pretty good strip.'

Skimming over the airstrip, the pilots spot crowds of villagers who have gathered to watch. 'Poor bastards,' Richard laughs. 'They think we're not going to land. Food? What food? We've brought no food.'

The plane circles the town and returns to the approach to the airstrip. 'Give me four flaps and override on HPR,' he orders. The Casa swoops, then roars as Richard jams it into reverse. 'Plus five, plus two, we're there,' he exclaims as the plane lands on the bumpy turf, sending a dog on the strip running for his life. 'Cheated death yet again.'

The entire village, it seems, has come to get a look at the *gringos*. Women with babies hanging from their breasts sell pawpaws and croquet-sized balls of raw chocolate. Young men help the agents pull crates of food from the plane's belly and load them onto ox carts. Most of the provisions are for the coast guard, but there are some for the village too following a request from the mayor. Favours like this are good PR. 'Once they even asked us to fly their soccer team here,' says Richard. Wilting in the mid-afternoon heat, the crowd slowly embarks on the mile-long trek through the village to the river.

True to its name, Bella Vista is one of the most tranquil places on earth. Its 100-odd inhabitants live from fishing, tropical fruits and cattle. Beef here costs less than a dollar a kilo. Since no-one has ever committed a crime, they have never bothered to build a police station.

The Americans drop off some dental kits at the largest house in the village, an orphanage run by a Spanish nun. Some villagers wave shyly. 'Last week we had a football match, villagers on one side, coast guard, DEA and UMOPAR on the other,' recalls one agent, plucking a grapefruit from a tree beside the path. 'Whoever won had to buy a cow for a barbecue. They beat the dog out of us.' But the villagers are less eager to play the game when it comes to speaking about drugs. If they talk, they fear they will be killed.

The group reaches the battered converted ferry, which will serve as home for the next three weeks. They call her the *Bolivian Queen*. Beside her are moored six inflatable Piranha patrol boats which will be used on tributaries too narrow for the mother ship. On the banks, the agents will hopefully find airstrips, cocaine stashes or labs that use the river water for processing. Recently, though, the traffickers have been hiding their operations away from the rivers to avoid the police. Then the agents have to 'infil'.

The Americans climb on board and sling their M-16s and packs onto their bunks on the upper deck. The dormitory is neat and clean, a contrast with the squalid UMOPAR quarters below. When they sleep, the agents cage themselves inside nets against the mosquitoes. 'At home you get mosquitos in threes and fours. Here they come in hundreds of thousands,' says one. 'You need air traffic control.'

Conditions are basic. The crew will live off pasta and tomato sauce, with meat every other day, prepared by the UMOPAR cook. It gets so hot the agents have to change their clothes three times a day. They swim off the boat, but have to be careful to avoid the piranhas.

Once afloat, the agents will stop at local communities in search of dope. They are forbidden by Bolivian law to enter homes, or to carry out arrests or interrogations. Instead, they hang around the local drinking hole and order beers in threes. 'They see you have money, so things begin to come out,' says an agent called Victor. 'You ask if there is an airstrip where you could land, or if there are any foreigners. Usually they don't say a word, they're too scared. So you look out for tell-tale signs like imported goods: a plastic spoon, a watch, exotic clothes, or a car. If you spot any of those you smell a rat.'

Communicating with the UMOPAR and navy guys can be equally difficult. Although all Snowcappers now attend language school before they come, few are fluent in Spanish apart from the Hispanics. 'There they teach you things like "How can I find a baby-sitter" or "Is there a good hotel here?" — not exactly the things you need to ask here,' says one agent.

There is resentment, too, stemming from the difference in salaries between the Americans and the Bolivians. 'The Bolivians do nothing but scrounge,' says a coast-guard agent called Pete.

They're like retarded children. They want everything we have. When I first arrived on the boat I told them: 'I smoke. I've got a packet of cigarettes. If you smoke you'd better get your own before we set off. Everyone has to pay for their own vices.' No-one asked me for a cigarette the whole time. America is like a big tit for them. They suck it till it goes dry, then they go running to the traffickers.

The only people Pete trusts are the other coast guards.

When they return from the river operation, the agents will hopefully bring back a kilo or two of cocaine and a few precursors. They may even have bust the odd lab. But none are under any illusion it will make much difference back home. 'It doesn't matter how many labs I destroy,' says Pete. 'Demand is the problem. I do this because it's a job and they sent me here.

I'd rather be at home with my kids and family. This job is costing me my marriage.' Another is more optimistic.

> We're winning some battles, although the war still has a long way to go. But at least I know that every lab I bust I am stopping one or two grammes of cocaine entering the US and poisoning my children and my friends' children. Put it this way: if we left, what would it be like? The police would probably be the main traffickers because they have the weapons. The traffickers would roam free. What we are doing may be the tip of the iceberg, but at least we're stopping things getting out of control.

ON THE morning of 14 July 1986, residents of Santa Cruz were woken by a roar of low-flying planes. Looking out of their windows, they noticed that the planes were not the usual Cessnas the traffickers flew into the airport every day. And they were substantially larger than the commercial Bolivian Air Lines jets that flew daily to and from La Paz and Miami. Looking closer they saw that the planes lumbering onto the tarmac included a Galaxy C-5A transport plane and two planes which looked like C-130s.

Nearly 200 neatly turned-out US troops in full combat gear spilled out of the C-130s. From the C-5A transport plane they unloaded six high-performance Black Hawk choppers. Then trucks, jeeps, radio equipment and ammunition. The *cruceños*, not usually easily impressed, had never seen anything like it.

Bolivian journalists who watched the Americans arrive rushed to their offices. Hysterical headlines in Santa Cruz newspapers next evening spoke of invasion. Reporters from the US and Europe jumped on the first planes to Santa Cruz. The international press had not gathered in such numbers in Bolivia since the death of Che Guevara.

The operation, codenamed Operation Blast Furnace, had been planned in the strictest secrecy for months. One of the largest international drug busts ever to be undertaken, it aimed to deal a mortal blow to Bolivia's traffickers. In particular, it hoped to destroy the business of one man the DEA had been hunting for years: Roberto Suárez.

Now, one day into the operation, the discreet international drug raid was fast turning into a public extravaganza. The US soldiers had not even had time to train their Bolivian counterparts. Apparently it had not occurred to the operation's Pentagon planners that it might be a bit difficult to conceal the arrival of a Galaxy cargo plane, six Black Hawk choppers, two support planes, 160 US troops, 20 DEA agents, and a fleet of assorted doctors, mechanics and communications experts.

It was not the first time a US-led drugs bust had gone public, of course. DEA agents were used to that. But this time they had hoped it would be different. 'It's all politics' grumbled a veteran drug war warrior. 'Every big operation we've had for the past two years... has been blown.'[5]

Secrecy (or lack of it) was not the only problem. The operation had already been delayed by three days because petrol workers in Santa Cruz had staged a wildcat strike. Pilots of the planes which were about to set out from Panama could not carry the 20,000 gallons of fuel they needed for the return trip. Not relishing the thought of their planes being stranded on the tarmac at the mercy of the traffickers, the pilots did not want to fly into Santa Cruz unless immediate refuelling could be guaranteed.

The operation had been conceived by DEA administrator Jack Lawn following talks with the Bolivians at a drug conference in Argentina. But the man who readied the troops for battle was Vice-President George Bush, then chairman of the National Narcotics Border Interdiction System, a task force set up in 1983 to streamline the fight against narcotics but which had achieved minimal results. He pressured the Pentagon into committing the Black Hawks, but only after a long battle with defense secretary, Caspar Weinberger, who believed the role of US troops was to defend their country from foreign attack, not to fight cocaine kingpins in the jungles of South America. It took a personal phone call from President Reagan, who had just signed a secret directive allowing US forces to fight drugs abroad, to win him over. There was dissent from other quarters too. The *Washington Post* saw it as yet another example of the administration focusing on foreign countries when the real problem was consumption in the US. 'American troops are where they do not belong, fighting a war on Bolivia that cannot even be won at home,' said feature-writer Richard Cohen. 'Usually it is truth that is war's first casualty. In the war on drugs it appears to be common sense.'

Operating out of a rear base in Trinidad and a forward base about 100 miles north, the bust aimed to destroy about 50 cocaine labs in the Beni which had previously been out of the reach of Bolivian police choppers. Almost a third were said to belong to Roberto Suárez. DEA agents knew there was no chance they would find the man himself. He would have been tipped off weeks in advance, probably by friends in the Interior Ministry, and would already be sampling the night clubs of Colombia or Brazil. But if they could throw his operations into temporary disarray, that would be something. 'Until then the traffickers had been relaxed because they knew we didn't have the means to tackle them,' recalls a Bolivian policeman. 'We needed the Americans to get them scared.'

Originally the DEA intended to send six of its men and asked the Pentagon to send some 20 troops to do maintenance. But somehow the operation mysteriously grew. The Pentagon decided it would send six planes and 89 men. On top of that it wanted doctors, mechanics, communications experts and so on. Soon the number of people had crept to 160. The DEA, which was now to send a mere 20 agents, was livid.

US politicians, who realised that drugs were now a top political issue, were in high spirits. They could now show that the US was getting tough. 'I approve of what the president did. We've got to go to the source of drugs,' said Tip O'Neil, the speaker of the house.[6] Bolivia's leaders, for their part, saw the operation as a useful way of cleaning up their drug-stained image and wiping out US doubts about their enthusiasm to tackle drugs. Feelings were admittedly running high against letting in US troops, but Bolivia's leaders hoped these would be compensated for by injections of US aid, which Bolivia desperately needed.

Pentagon planners had another reason to be pleased. Now they had convinced Bolivia, traditionally the pariah of the world drugs trade, to allow US troops and DEA agents to help fight drug trafficking, there was hope they might be able to persuade other countries, like Mexico and Colombia, to follow suit. Technically, of course, the troops would not play an active role and were merely 'technicians'. But they would set an important precedent.

With the cover blown, some DEA agents wondered if they should go ahead with the operation. They decided it was just worth it. But they knew its value would be more symbolic than real.

For the next four months, US troops and Bolivian Leopards were flown by US pilots into the heart of cocaine country. They raided laboratories, dynamited airstrips and confiscated chemicals, aeroplanes and documents.

Their first bust was a lab about 60 miles north of their staging base known as El Zorro (The Fox). The site had two airstrips, and 15 large camouflaged tents housing about 75 workers. There was a restaurant, a children's playground and a basketball court. The lab had been manufacturing 700 kilos of cocaine a week. When the Leopards arrived, however, no-one was at home. The lab had been dismantled and all that remained were a couple of barrels of gasolene and some chemicals. Not a gramme of drugs. Villagers later told police that the inhabitants of El Zorro had fled several days earlier after being tipped off.

Suddenly the Leopards heard the sound of the engine of a small plane. A Cessna landed on one of the airstrips and a man and a boy got out. When he realised who the visitors were the pilot fled into the jungle, leaving his 17-year-old assistant to explain himself. The youth said his job was to wash planes. The Leopards seized the Cessna and bundled the boy into the chopper — their first captive.

Later that week, the Leopards targeted a remote camp in the Department of La Paz with a 1,600-metre airstrip. This time the results were even more disappointing. All the agents found were bemused *campesinos* tending their cattle and tilling their fields.

In September the US decided to tackle Santa Ana, which is a major trafficking centre and outside the government's control. But the 80 Bolivians and 30 Americans who carried out the raid were forced to flee after a 3,000-

strong mob shouting 'Kill the Yankees' pursued them with machetes. They made no arrests and found no drugs.

But the security forces made one extraordinary omission: Huanchaca, a vast 'drive-in' cocaine hydrochloride lab near Santa Cruz reportedly owned by Techo de Paja or the Chavez family. The Americans apparently knew about the lab and had even photographed it, but failed to act until Noel Kempff, the director of the Santa Cruz Botanical and Zoological Garden, was machine-gunned to death by traffickers a few weeks later while collecting specimens. Even then, Bolivian and US security forces took 47 hours to reach it, two hours more than the families of the dead men, by which time the traffickers had long fled. To many Bolivians it looked like a cover-up. Despite official inquiries, the truth has never been established. An investigator called Edmundo Salazar, who announced he was about to make 'sensational revelations' about Huanchaca, was assassinated a few hours later. One Bolivian account maintained that the lab was run by the CIA to raise money for US-backed Contras attempting to overthrow the Nicaraguan government. The theory is denied by US officials, but controversy over Huanchaca continues to this day.

Blast Furnace had some short-term successes. The price of the coca leaf had slumped from $125 to between $10 and $20 a *carga*. Chapare farmers who had no-one to sell to were queuing up for seeds to grow alternative crops. *Campesinos* who had worked at the laboratories as cooks, cleaners or technicians flocked into the cities to look for employment.

Arrests and seizures, however, were disappointing. Only one person was arrested (the 17-year-old) and virtually no cocaine was found. Only 21 labs had been destroyed, a tiny number given the resources pitted against them.

Operation Dope, as its critics dubbed it, was clearly not quite the glittering success intended. The Bolivians blamed the US. 'If US technology is capable of hitting the house of Colonel Gaddafi without damaging neighbouring houses, how is it possible that they can't find cocaine laboratories in Bolivia?' asked one Bolivian newspaper commentator. In Washington, though, politicians were not ready to concede defeat. Operation Blast Furnace, said Reagan, had been a 'big success' even though there had been a 'few mistakes'. Asked to explain why the operation had achieved so few results, White House aides declared that its success had been above all psychological. 'There is no clear victory in an operation like this,' declared one Bush aide. 'This is not Grenada.'[7]

The US could not wage the Bolivians' war for them forever. 'They were desperate to go back,' says a Bolivian politician. 'They were scared stiff someone was going to get hurt.' On 25 October a C5-A transport plane lifted off from Santa Cruz airport with three Black Hawks. Three weeks later the other three Black Hawks left with over 100 US military personnel. The traffickers, who had been in hiding in Bolivia or Brazil while the operation had been under way, sprang back to life. As soon as the date of the

Americans' departure had been announced, they began buying coca leaves again in preparation for the reopening of their paralysed labs. By October the price of leaves was double that of a month earlier. For those whose operations had survived intact, Operation Blast Furnace had had the added benefit of wiping out competition. Now with only the Bolivian police to deal with, business was going to boom.

WHILE US troops had been ferrying Bolivian police through the jungles of the Beni, their bosses in Washington had been meeting to discuss where Operation Blast Furnace had gone wrong and what lessons could be learned.

One thing was clear: if interdiction was to work it had to be long-term. A short-term offensive might be moderately effective while it lasted but once the pressure was off things would simply return to normal. But a long-term offensive on the scale of Blast Furnace was impossible because of its cost in resources and manpower.

Another problem was that the high visibility of US troops during the operation had aroused strong anti-US feeling in Bolivia and neighbouring South American countries. 'Despite its success,' admitted David Westrate, the DEA's assistant administrator, 'the high visibility of US military operations in Bolivia [was] extremely controversial and the operation was short lived.'[8] What was needed, officials argued, was a long-term operation in which US military personnel would play a vital but discreet role. The outcome was Operation Snowcap.

Although no-one knew at the time, the C5-A transport planes which collected the Blast Furnace troops and equipment brought with them six UH-1 Huey helicopters and a US army Snowcap training team. This time the DEA and the Pentagon would succeed in avoiding the catastrophic publicity that had almost ruined Blast Furnace. No public announcement of Snowcap was ever made. Even today some elements of the programme, including its overall cost and the number of agents involved, remain classified. When the media did talk about it, Snowcap officials were careful to play down the operation. 'We tried to arrange the profile in such away that it is perfectly acceptable politically, media-wise and every other way in support of what we are trying to do,' declared Westrate.[9] Snowcap's aim, he said, was to cut the amount of cocaine entering the US by half over three years. Hundreds of Snowcap agents were sent to risk their lives in the three main Andean cocaine-producer countries. The DEA put all its eggs into the Snowcap basket. As one DEA agent put it at the time, 'If [Snowcap] doesn't work, [the DEA] is down the tubes. Within the federal law enforcement community and with Congress, Snowcap was sold up and down the Potomac. Snowcap may not be the best game in town, but it's the only game. It has to be successful, one way or the other.'[10]

THREE YEARS later, the period within which Snowcap was supposed to have achieved its aims, seizures had indeed increased dramatically. Success was measured in terms of kilos of coke confiscated and airstrips blown to pieces. Sensational large raids, which hit the media headlines, were used as proof that America's drugs war was being won. In 1990, as cocaine prices in some parts of the US soared and purity dropped, officials began to talk of victory. 'We are finally making progress in the international war against cocaine', declared Westrate in May 1990.[11] 'The traffickers are hunted men.'

What Westrate and other officials failed to mention was that although seizures were up, cocaine production was soaring even faster. Snowcap had fallen way short of its aim of slashing the supply of cocaine to the US by half. 'The goal of reducing cocaine availability in the US has not been met,' said a 1990 congressional report on Snowcap. 'In fact, cocaine availability has increased dramatically since 1983.' In Bolivia, it said, narcotics inter- diction efforts in 1989 had been 'infrequent and generally ineffective'. Having spent millions of dollars of US tax-payers' money, Snowcap had seized one half of 1 per cent of Bolivia's estimated cocaine hydrochloride and base production.[12]

In Washington, though, DEA officials were determined to put a brave face on things. Their attitude is exemplified in an exchange between Westrate and Congressman Benjamin Gilman (Republican: New York) during hearings before the House Foreign Affairs Committee in 1990:[13]

Gilman: What have we reached at this point, what reductions since you started?

Westrate: Well, the production has not reduced at all really yet. But I think what we are seeing...

Gilman [interrupting]: Has there been any reduction in supply?

Westrate: What we are seeing is a lot of disruption. And I think that there are a lot of signs out there.

Gilman: I know that you are disrupting, and I know that you are interdicting, and I know that you are raiding, but I'm asking you, Mr Westrate, has there been any reduction in supply?

Westrate: I cannot say at this point...

Westrate assured his interrogator that Snowcap was at a 'turning point'. It just needed a few more years to work. Meanwhile, Snowcap had adjusted its goal to reducing the influx of cocaine by half within ten years instead of three.

Congressmen like Larry Smith (Democrat: Florida) were unimpressed. 'It is very hard to continue to try to feel the commitment to these programmes when the results are extremely disappointing,' he told Westrate at the same hearing. 'After three years of the US providing a significant amount of money we have not seen a significant amount of return for the kind of investment that has been made.'

Mike Levine, the DEA under-cover agent who had masterminded the sting operation against Roberto Suárez, now retired and making a living writing books about his experiences, took an even dimmer view. He said the notion of success lying 'just around the corner', first used by Reagan, was one of the favourite inside DEA jokes which never failed to get a laugh among the Washington 'suits' (bureaucrats). He claimed that the DEA knew that it had failed but was trying to cover it up. 'The drug war is a fraud,' he claimed in an interview.[14]

> Every drug enforcement agent knows that what you read in the press has nothing to do with what's really happening.... By eradicating crops and destroying labs through military intervention, the US will defend its shores against the influx of the white death — that's the media version. In point of fact, I was told by... one of the people running Snowcap, that the operation was a sham. 'We know this programme doesn't work.... Congress asked us, what is our answer to the cocaine war? It's Operation Snowcap. It will succeed one way or the other.'

Despite the DEA's hope that by destroying cocaine labs they will drive coca farmers out of business, this has not happened. The area planted with coca in Bolivia increased by 10 per cent between 1988 and 1989 and has since remained more or less level. Although the price of the leaf in Bolivia and Peru dropped to an unprecedented low in early 1990, by 1991 it had returned to very profitable levels, repeating historical patterns of price fluctuations.

Critics believe Operation Snowcap simply ignores laws of supply and demand. In the short term, interdiction efforts targeted at big cocaine labs may disrupt operations and push up the price of cocaine. But because there is always US demand, there will always be the refiners, exporters and smugglers willing to risk getting cocaine to the US or Europe. When disrupted they simply move deeper into the jungle, out of range of US helicopters, or even into new countries, where they will be harassed less. 'Every time we disrupt or close a particular trafficking route, we have found that traffickers resort to other smuggling tactics that are even more difficult to detect,' admitted a 1989 report by President Bush.

When the DEA arrived in Trinidad, for example, the traffickers simply moved deeper into the Beni, outside the 100-mile radius covered by the US Hueys. 'Every trafficker has maps marking the radius of the DEA choppers. They set up their labs outside it,' says a DEA agent. A game of cat and mouse followed, as the DEA tried to extend its range by setting up a Forward Operating Base at Primavera, 110 miles north, and the traffickers moved even further afield. In the end, though, the area of Amazon jungle into which traffickers can move their operations is virtually limitless. In the process, they slash more and more rain forest and pollute more and more rivers. With their vast resources, they can set up new labs and trafficking routes within weeks.

Some US economists say that even if eradication efforts in the Andean countries did manage to lower cocaine prices, this would have virtually no effect on the price in the US. This is because most of the profits are added at the final link of the chain, i.e. distribution in the US. A study by the Rand Corporation showed that in 1986 a kilo of cocaine at the farm was worth $1,200. On export from Colombia after processing, it was worth $7,000, rocketing to $20,000 on arrival at Miami. Wholesale in Detroit the price doubled. By the time the cocaine was sold on the street it was worth an astronomical $250,000. Law enforcement at the Andean end, the economists concluded, was virtually useless. It was on the streets of the US that action needed to be taken.

Critics of Snowcap say it is not only failing to achieve its aims but is also exposing its agents to unnecessary danger. DEA agents, trained to work on the streets of US cities, are being forced to carry out paramilitary activities in a jungle environment with which they are totally unfamiliar. 'There's a fundamental mismatch here. You've got street cops from Cincinnati trying to fight a war in the jungle,' declared US Ambassador Robert Gelbard in 1989. 'We have to take a really fresh look at what we are doing.'[15] According to a 1989 Department of State Inspector-General audit, many DEA agents at that time could not speak Spanish and the only military training most received was a two-week jungle survival course. Training was later upgraded to 12 weeks of jungle warfare training from the US Special Forces at Fort Benning, Georgia, and five weeks tactical training from the Marine Corps. Even then, many believed that was hardly enough to equip them to take on some of the world's most violent criminals in one of the most hostile environments on earth.

Only one Snowcapper has so far been killed. He was Rick Finley, who died, along with eight non-DEA people, in an aeroplane crash in Peru's Upper Huallaga Valley, where most Peruvian coca is grown. In Bolivia, DEA agents narrowly escaped being massacred when they were caught in cross-fire in ,1990. Many agents believe it is only a matter of time before more die, particularly in countries like Peru where traffickers or growers are defended by Maoist Shining Path guerrillas. The starkest warning came from Frank White, chief of DEA special training, in 1988. In a secret memo, leaked to the press, he warned that without immediate changes 'DEA agents are going to agonise alone through an excruciating death on an isolated jungle floor'. When Snowcap increased the number of personnel in Bolivia in 1988, a top DEA official warned that the Snowcap operations were a 'path to disaster'.[16] Agents were being sent with little or no training, poor leadership and shoddy equipment, and none of the DEA or State Department bureaucrats seemed to care. Rumours circulated in the DEA that large quantities of bodybags were among the equipment being sent to South

America. 'It makes your blood run cold,' warned another drugs official. 'At what point did we decide that the DEA should be fighting in the jungles of South America?... We've backed into this and nobody's thought this through at the highest levels of this government.'[17]

A congressional report by the House Foreign Affairs Committee's Task Force on International Narcotics in 1989 was equally critical. '[The] DEA is being thrust into essentially a paramilitary role for which it is ill-equipped [and] the [Bureau for] International Narcotics Matters [which supplies the DEA with air support] is operating an air wing for which it has no expertise,' it said. It also expressed concern over the fact that no evacuation plans existed for US personnel in dangerous environments, and that assault helicopters had no defensive weapons.

Officials in Washington had a range of different solutions to Snowcap's clear failure. Some believed it would never succeed, however well trained the US agents, because the forces of Andean countries were so hopelessly corrupt or because the basic problem was US demand. Others, like Johnstone, believed Snowcap could make an impact, but only if it had more resources. At present, he says, Congress appears to expect results but is unwilling to grant the money and materials that the operation needs. 'With three helicopters we are supposed to cover an area the size of New Jersey,' he says. 'How can we possibly achieve anything?' To be effective, he believes he would need 30 helicopters and twice as many agents.

Others wanted a more aggressive stance against the Latin druglords. People like General Thurman, former head of the Southern Command in Panama, wanted an all-out war, rather than what they saw as polite pussy-footing. They wanted DEA agents replaced by US Special Forces personnel better trained for the paramilitary operations being carried out by DEA agents. '[DEA agents] are cops' an officer on Thurman's staff was quoted as saying. 'Very brave, but cops.'[18] In Thurman's view, cops were for collaring criminals on the street, not masterminding the overthrow of international cartels. Many members of the US Congress agreed. 'Let's push this damn thing,' said Congressman Nicholas Mavroules in 1989. 'We can't stop them [drug dealers] without the military.'

US Special Forces had maintained a discreet presence in Bolivia since 1987, training Bolivian police and providing support for the DEA. In his September 1989 Andean Initiative, President Bush signalled they were now to become a major force in the 'war' against drugs in the Andes, helping in areas like intelligence gathering, planning and training. Some officials believed their involvement would eventually pave the way for the DEA to pull out. A report in 1990 said the DEA was preparing a phased withdrawal, but it was promptly denied by DEA officials, keen to defend their institution from an encroaching Department of Defense.

Other US Special Forces are being used to train Andean armies that have been drawn into the drugs fight. In Bolivia, 56 US military advisers were sent to train two battalions of the Bolivian army. They started in 1991 at the headquarters of Bolivia's Ranger Battalion at Montero, 60 miles north of Santa Cruz, which was established in the 1960s by the US to fight Che Guevara. They later moved to Riberalta, in the northern Beni.

US officials insist that US military personnel will not accompany Bolivian forces on operations, as DEA agents had done. Overall, they appear to have observed those rules. 'We go as far as we can with the military short of actually taking them on operations,' says a DEA agent. One former US embassy employee who served in Bolivia from 1985 to 1987, however, reported that Special Forces agents accompanied Bolivian forces on operations at the completion of training programmes.[19]

None the less, there are fears that they may get sucked into combat situations. In 1989 President Bush is reported to have signed a secret National Security Directive changing the rules of engagement so that Special Forces could accompany their foreign trainees on 'training missions' in areas considered 'secure'. Although the guidelines were designed to limit US involvement, in practice they were meaningless since there was no guarantee that traffickers and guerrillas would refrain from attacking simply because a patrol was a training patrol or because it was in a supposedly 'safe' area. In any case, according to one report by US Special Forces, like DEA 'advisers', US military personnel often see such rules as bureaucratic niceties in the hostile environment of the Andean jungle. 'There are lots of ways to get killed down here, and our best survivors here are the Green Berets,' a Special Operations staff officer at Southcom was quoted as saying. 'It only makes common sense to let them go on combat missions with their newly trained and equipped drug teams. School is one thing. These jungles are another.'[20]

Whether they are advisers or combat troops, critics of Washington's drugs policy believe that any visible presence of US military personnel could put them at extreme risk. 'The mere presence of US units in the volatile Andean region creates the prospect of their being caught in the crossfire between the druglords and government forces,' says Ted Carpenter, director of the Cato Institute, a Washington think tank. 'In that case, US military involvement could easily escalate for "defensive" reasons.' If US personnel were attacked, who would they retaliate against? 'You're chasing clouds, you're chasing nothing,' says CRS military analyst Robert Goldich.[21] 'And at that point, the US public will look and say what are we getting out of this? And will become intensely frustrated, completely understandably, because when we are hit there appears to be no way to hit back.'

The military were useful for the equipment and cash they provided, but many DEA agents in Bolivia resented them in much the same way that UMOPAR resent the involvement of the Bolivian military. Many agents felt they were quite capable of doing their job and felt that military personnel who had not made it at home were being palmed off on them. 'Many of the guys we got were dead beat,' says one. The atmosphere was tense and there were repeated squabbles between the two institutions as both defended their turfs. On several occasions the DEA was unable to get help from the Department of Defense personnel to transport equipment to DEA agents in the field.[22] Inter-agency bickering undermined the training of Bolivian police, according to a report by the Department of State inspector general. The Leopards, for example, were trained by US army Special Forces in jungle survival, military operations and small-unit tactics. But because Special Forces were prohibited from accompanying them on missions, the Leopards were then turned over to DEA agents who taught them different military tactics which, according to one Special Forces officer, were dangerous and defeated the purpose of training.[23]

DEA officials also believe that the military is inappropriate in a war with no front line and no neatly grouped enemy. It is like trying to swat mosquitoes with a sledge-hammer. As one put it: 'The CIA and the military have spent ten years trying to find one goddam hostage in Lebanon. What makes them think they can come down [to South America] and solve the dope problem?'[24] The military are trained to seek out and destroy an enemy in wartime, not in the nuances of law enforcement, which in the US has always been a civilian concern. 'The military's answer is to blow everyone up,' says the DEA's Gene Castillo.

> They call this a 'war' on drugs. It is a war of sorts, but it is still a law enforcement operation which has to be carried out according to the laws of the country we are in. Often I'd like to just go and get rid of a crook. But you can't do it that way. He has rights and we can't just go and violate them. We have to arrest him and produce proof, not just kill him. Even under a dictatorship we cannot do things this way. We are still, hopefully, a civilised country and have to respect laws.

Another DEA agent, a pilot who did a year in Vietnam, agrees. 'People back home say "Why don't you nuke the bad guys?" I say "We can't do that, we're in someone else's country."'

8

Walking the Tightrope:
The Politicians

La Paz

IN LA PAZ on the morning of 25 February 1991 the telephone rang in the plush sixth-floor embassy office of Bob Gelbard, the US ambassador. Gelbard grabbed the phone while skimming through the morning's cables.

'Hello, Gelbard,' he said.[1]

'Hello ambassador, it's Faustino Rico Toro here,' said the voice on the other end in Spanish. 'I've just been appointed to head the Special Force for the Fight Against Drug Trafficking.'

Gelbard couldn't believe his ears. He grunted, searching for something to say.

'I'd like to meet for a chat,' continued the voice on the other end.

'I'm sorry,' replied Gelbard. 'I'm terribly busy. I'm about to leave for Santa Cruz. I am going to visit the High Valleys development project with some Bolivian journalists.' He slammed the phone down.

Gelbard was stunned. Rico Toro was known to be a close friend of García Meza, and the DEA had more than a dozen cases dating from the early 1980s reputedly implicating him in the cocaine trade. Both Arce Gómez and García Meza had almost certainly hidden in ranches owned by Rico Toro, and García Meza might still be there. The man also had an appalling human rights record. As chief of a secret army intelligence unit during García Meza's regime, he had allegedly supervised death squads which tortured and murdered scores of political opponents. Incidentally, he had picked up his intelligence skills in Florida where he had been sent on a training course during the military regime of General Barrientos in the 1960s when catching commies was the game of the day. Later he had become a close friend of Klaus Barbie, who had been a regular visitor to Rico Toro's Section Two office. Putting him in charge of the Special Force

163

was, as one labour leader put it, 'like asking a cat to look after a can of sardines'.

Gelbard had to get the appointment annulled before Rico Toro was officially sworn in. If it got to that stage a head-on clash between the government and the US embassy would be inevitable.

Gelbard called a couple of people in the Bolivian government whom he could trust, then caught his plane.

Next morning a call was put through to Gelbard's Santa Cruz hotel room from Gonzálo Torrico, the under-secretary for social defence in the Interior Ministry. He was ringing, he said, on the orders of the interior minister, Guillermo Capobianco, to find out what Gelbard thought of the Rico Toro appointment. Gelbard replied that it was the decision of a sovereign Bolivian government but added that the man's murky record both in fighting drugs and in respecting human rights would give him 'extreme difficulty' in accepting it. Later that morning he tried to phone Capobianco himself but was fobbed off by a secretary who said he was 'unavailable'. Capobianco was clearly anxious to avoid a fight until he'd got Rico Toro sworn in.

Capobianco, a close friend of the president, was well aware of the strength of feeling against Rico Toro. But far from holding him back, it goaded him on. This time Capobianco was determined not to let the *gringos* have things their way. He brought forward the swearing-in session. By the night of 26 February Rico Toro, an alleged drugs trafficker, was head of Bolivia's US-funded Special Force for the Fight Against Drug Trafficking.

There was uproar in Bolivia. General Banzer, the head of the ADN party which was a co-member of the coalition government and, as a military man, someone who knew more than most about Rico Toro's past, had not been consulted and was furious. In fact it was his party that had given Rico Toro his previous job of president of the Cochabamba Development Corporation (CORDECO). The commander of the armed forces was also upset and stressed that the armed forces had nothing to do with the appointment. Some members of the cabinet opposed it. The widow of the Socialist deputy, Marcelo Quiroga Santa Cruz, murdered on the day of García Meza's coup, claimed that Rico Toro had been responsible for her husband's killing and was probably one of the few who knew where his body was.

The biggest mystery was how President Paz could have made such a colossal misjudgement as to appoint a man who was universally loathed. One explanation (the US one) was that the appointment had been foisted on Paz by Capobianco and was part of a carefully worked out plan to give the drug traffickers a free hand. Another was that the government had got so fed up with being bossed around by the US that it believed Rico Toro, who had been currying favour with Jaime Paz and his cronies, would be the best man to sort them out.

Another explanation was that the appointment was what is known in Bolivia as a *historia de faldas* (a skirts affair). Rico Toro happened to have an exceedingly beautiful daughter. She had even been a finalist in the Miss Universe contest. Jaime Paz had been photographed dancing in the streets with her at carnival time and, it was rumoured, was completely smitten. What better way to bid for her affections than to give her father one of the highest profile posts in Bolivia? Over the previous months Rico Toro had on several occasions been seen at Jaime Paz's ranch. In return he had reportedly given the president a horse. Whatever the truth, it was, in the words of one US official, 'one bitch of a way to run a government'.

For Gelbard, Rico Toro's appointment was simply the last straw. Since taking power in the autumn of 1989, the government had shown minimal interest in fighting drugs. US officials had been incensed when immediately on taking office Paz appointed a number of corrupt officials to key anti-narcotics posts, and even more so when, confronted by Gelbard, Paz had allegedly responded that 'since most police were corrupt it didn't matter anyway'.[2] When the US ambassador insisted, the government had replaced the officials, but six months later had brought in another corrupt batch, many of whom had worked for the García Meza regime and later been sacked for drugs trafficking. By appointing Rico Toro, the government showed that it apparently no longer cared. This was two fingers to US anti-narcotics efforts in Bolivia.

In the past US diplomats would have sat and smarted, putting a show of smooth relations before the fight against drugs. But Gelbard was of a different school. Drugs came at the top of his agenda, even when that conflicted with diplomacy. And he was a man who didn't mind saying what he thought. As one Bolivian politician who has dealt with Gelbard for many years put it, 'he is frank and brutal but at least he is up-front'. Gelbard was also backed by a bullish US president who had made drugs his number one priority. Diplomacy in Bolivia had changed accordingly. 'In the past we got ministers after the event, like Arce Gómez. Now we go and get them while they are still in place,' explained one US official.

To make it worse, Capobianco and other key ministers were unrepentant. 'The appointment of the commander of the special force is an exercise of national sovereignty. We reject the criticism,' the minister of information Mario Rueda told the Associated Press. 'We know what we are doing,' declared Jaime Paz lamely, despite the fact that he clearly did not. 'People are stuck in the past, they are chained to the past.'

That same week the State Department was releasing its annual report on the international drugs situation. Ironically it certified Bolivia as 'fully cooperating', noting that Bolivia had succeeded in meeting that year's coca eradication target. With an alleged drugs trafficker in charge of Bolivia's war against drugs, the report was going to look a little bit stupid.

After consulting with Washington, Gelbard rang two cabinet ministers to tell them that $120 million of US aid to Bolivia was now frozen. 'This raises serious questions about Bolivia's ability to handle anti-narcotics in a serious way,' he told the *Miami Herald* on 4 March 1991. 'In the light of these events we are carefully examining our ability to do business with the Bolivian government.' Another US official went further. 'We cannot deal with this man, and we're not going to,' he said. 'He's one of the most notorious people in Bolivia's recent history.'

Privately, Gelbard had been engaged in intensive discussions with 'friendly' members of the government. Ironically, his main ally was Banzer, under whose dictatorship the cocaine industry had taken off in earnest. Now, as the leader of the other party in government and a counterbalance to what Gelbard saw as Paz's distasteful ideological tendencies, Banzer was a useful friend. The pair spent two hours discussing the matter on Friday 1 March. Later that day, Banzer called Paz at the presidential palace. 'I have to see you,' he said. Paz said he was busy but Banzer insisted, and went straight to the palace. 'You have to get Rico Toro to resign immediately,' Banzer told the president. Paz stalled. He wasn't willing to carry out the dirty work of asking a close personal friend to resign, but if Banzer would do it, that was OK. They agreed that Banzer and the leader of Paz's Revolutionary Leftist Movement (MIR) party, Oscar Eid, would fly to Santa Cruz on the Monday morning to demand Rico Toro's resignation.

On Monday 4 March the news became public that Rico Toro had stepped down. Capobianco immediately accepted it but gave no explanation. Privately, MIR officials admitted that the Rico Toro appointment had been a disastrous mistake on the part of a dithering president who didn't seem even to know his own mind. 'We didn't expect the Americans to react so strongly. We simply miscalculated,' admitted one senior aide. Washington, quietly delighted, unfroze its aid.

But the affair could not end there. The ball that the Bolivians had sent the US was so hard that Gelbard was determined to return it. If the government was going to abandon all pretence of fighting drugs, he too was going to abandon all pretence that government officials were not involved in the game. Subtlety clearly did not work. In the words of one US official: 'We had reached a point of no return with the Bolivians.' It was time to clean the slate once and for all. Gelbard was ready to name names.

He chose Capobianco.

A handsome silver-haired 38-year-old, Capobianco had been an MIR party militant for 20 years and was a close friend of the president. Paz had sealed their friendship by giving Capobianco the ministry he most wanted, the Interior. But the US embassy had suspicions about him and had been watching him carefully. Before taking office Capobianco had reportedly introduced Paz to one of Bolivia's biggest drugs traffickers, Isaac Chavarría, who US sources say contributed substantial funds and the use of several private aeroplanes to Paz's election campaign. As interior minister, Capobianco was responsible for choosing who should fill key departmental police commander positions. US officials were certain that Capobianco was behind the appointment of the latest batch of allegedly corrupt officers. They were also sure that, like many an interior minister before him, Capobianco was receiving payoffs from some important drug barons. Although from a humble family, he had mysteriously acquired a $4 million ranch. When he visited his home city of Santa Cruz, the car that sometimes collected him belonged to Chavarría.

As his medium, Gelbard selected the *Miami Herald*. He rang Sam Dillon, the paper's correspondent in Santiago, and leaked devastating corruption allegations against Capobianco. He also hit out against Felipe Carvajal, the National Police commander, who, it was claimed, had reinstated 40 police officers who had previously been sacked for drugs trafficking. In the story published in the *Miami Herald* on 4 March 1991, 'US officials' were quoted as saying that both had 'until recently been receiving payments from top Bolivian drugs organisations but have been hurt by recent anti-narcotics round-ups organised by DEA agents'. Rico Toro's appointment, the story said, had been part of a wider campaign by Capobianco and Carvajal to appoint compliant police officers who would cooperate with the traffickers. 'We've seen a systematic attempt on the part of these guys to appoint corrupt officials to key jobs in narcotics areas,' the 'US official' said. In the outcry that followed, the US embassy denied that Gelbard had spoken to the *Miami Herald* and did not know who had. Asked for evidence to substantiate their allegations, US officials declared they had passed evidence to the relevant Cabinet members but that it had not been necessary to make it public.

Bolivian politicians were furious and relations with the embassy slumped to an all-time low. With a single press article, Capobianco's career and reputation had been ruined. Was it really based on hard evidence? If so, why did the US refuse to divulge it? Perhaps there was none and the whole affair was a character assassination, grounded in the embassy's growing dislike for Paz's leftist government, and most recently his refusal to support the war against Saddam Hussein. Capobianco described the accusations as 'absolutely false, an infamous lie' which had 'damaged not only me, but my country, my president, and Bolivia's struggle against narcotics trafficking' and threatened to sue the *Miami Herald*. He was backed by the president who described the article as an 'outrage against the country' and declared his utmost faith in Capobianco's 'human and civic integrity'.

Many Bolivians, particularly those on the left, believed the episode was an outrageous intrusion by the US into the affairs of a foreign country. If Washington had the right to hire and fire Bolivia's ministers, then it was effectively running the country. US officials dismissed the accusations with characteristic vigour. 'They talk about sovereignty, but we're a sovereign country too', said one. 'By exporting cocaine they're violating our sovereignty.' Anti-imperialist sentiment became so heated that it began to eclipse any other considerations, like whether Capobianco was in fact guilty. No-one even suggested launching an investigation.

A few days after the *Miami Herald* article, Gelbard went out drinking with Jaime Paz to talk the matter over. In general, Gelbard did not consider Jaime a man of particularly high intellectual calibre, but the one thing they did share was football. Both were passionate about it. They started off discussing the latest match. Then, as their tongues were loosened by beer, they moved onto the subject that was bugging them both. 'You have to get rid of Capobianco and Carvajal,' said Gelbard. Paz was reluctant. He offered a compromise. He would sack Carvajal at once, but he would wait until August to deal with Capobianco. By then he would have been one year in office and a Cabinet reshuffle would not cause any great surprise. But Gelbard was not satisfied. He had only three months left as ambassador and wanted to go feeling he had left a clean slate. 'You have to get rid of Capobianco before I go,' he said. Paz said he would think about it.

For a while, Bolivian officials struggled on, adamantly defending Capobianco's reputation. But deep in their hearts they knew from bitter past experience that small underdeveloped countries like Bolivia do not win battles against a power like the US.

Gelbard did not even have to wait a week. Apart from anything else, Bolivia desperately needed US economic aid. A few days after Gelbard and Paz's late night session, Capobianco sent Paz his resignation letter in which he claimed that 'dark forces had been at work' but that his honour remained intact. He dropped his legal case against the *Miami Herald*. Government officials put a brave face on it saying that Capobianco would continue to serve the party in Santa Cruz. But US officials saw the rapidity of his resignation, and the fact that he had not really stood up for himself, as 'proof' that he had indeed been guilty of involvement in the drugs trade. 'A man, if he is innocent, fights longer than Capobianco did. And the president would have defended him to the end. That was not the case with Capobianco,' said one US official. Six months later Capobianco's younger brother, Luis 'Chichi' Capobianco gave himself up under a government decree allowing traffickers to avoid extradition to the US if they surrendered.

Two days later Carvajal went too, although the event passed virtually unnoticed amid the turmoil over Capobianco. The following month six high-ranking police officers were removed for corruption or incompetence.

CORRUPTION in the government, and US concern about it, was nothing new. For hundreds of years paying bribes has been the way to get things done in Bolivia, whether this meant paying off the customs man at the border to smuggle in an imported Mercedes, pulling strings to get one's cousin a job in a government ministry, or paying a judge to let one off a gaol sentence. Here, in the poorest country in South America, honesty is a luxury reserved for those able to afford it. The rules are well known by foreign companies who operate in Bolivia: to win a contract you pay off the relevant official. Bolivia, of course, is not unique in this respect, as the scandal surrounding the Bank of Credit and Commerce International in 1991 showed. It would be impossible to find a country in the world where corruption does not exist to a certain degree, including the US and Britain. Corruption in Bolivia is simply less sophisticated. Things are done the 'Latin way'.

When cocaine arrived on the scene in the late 1970s, things rapidly deteriorated. 'It was not a great leap to move from normal corruption to drugs corruption,' says a US official. As the industry was illicit, payoffs had to be made at every stage, especially as its organisation became more complex. The traffickers were so rich they could pay fantastic sums to buy off anyone who stood in their way. The stakes rose still higher as the barons increased their profits by making their own cocaine hydrochloride.

At first payoffs were *ad hoc*. But under the García Meza regime they developed into a complex 'formalised' system of corruption extending from Chapare paste buyers to cabinet ministers in La Paz. Drug enforcement experts believe the same system is still in place in Bolivia today, with the difference that politicians are now passive rather than active participants.

The system is like a pyramid. Each man pays off the man above him, usually through an intermediary, and that man in turn pays the guy above. The higher you go the higher the kickback.

At the bottom of the pyramid, traffickers from the various Mafias pay off the local police chief to allow them to smuggle in chemicals or land a small plane. He pays a percentage to his superior, the regional police commander, who in turn funnels money upwards to the national head of police. According to Western intelligence sources, the chief of police pays a percentage to the interior minister, who passes on some of the funds even higher, in other words to the president.

Not all traffickers conform to this system. Some make payoffs directly, though still via an intermediary, to key government ministers, such as the ministers of defence or the interior. The payoff is not necessarily paid as a crude cash sum. More often it is disguised as a contribution to the minister's party funds or election campaign, or paid into a company as a 'business deal'. According to Western intelligence sources, payoffs are sometimes made directly to the president.

When Paz's government took office, corruption allegedly grew rapidly worse. This was partly because there were now two parties in the Patriotic Accord coalition, the right-wing ADN party, headed by Hugo Banzer, and the left-wing MIR party, headed by Paz. This meant bribes of all types had to be paid twice over. They were expensive times for drugs traffickers.

Another reason was that the MIR had been in the political wilderness for 20 years and was now hungry for the privileges that go with power. As one US official put it, 'The MIR were like a bunch of broken-down lefties coming in from the cold. They said "Hey, it's raining soup. Get yourselves a bucket".'

Foreign companies began to feel the pinch. According to one US official, companies were told that if they wanted to do business it would help if they paid a 10 per cent commission on the value of the contract. Sometimes they were asked for even more. 'Corruption, far from diminishing, is increasing,' admitted the president of the Bolivian Confederation of Private Industries.

For US narcotics experts, who were now investing more time, energy and money in the war on drugs than ever before, corruption was their biggest headache. However much money they put into combating the drug barons, it was useless if police or government ministers were protecting them. Every time corrupt officials were appointed, the embassy complained and insisted they be replaced with men of their choosing. It was like a game of chess: every time the government made a move, the embassy made another, then the government made another.

The roots of the Rico Toro and Capobianco affair, however, lay in a raid UMOPAR and the DEA had carried out the previous September. Dubbed one of the most successful raids in Bolivian history, it was to prove a turning point in the battle over corruption.

AT 6.00 a.m. one September morning in 1990, a bus load of rowdy secondary school students hurtled along the road from Chimoré to Santa Cruz. Villagers along the way who heard their lewd songs and saw their blue and white school flags waving out of the windows imagined they were on a school outing or on the way to a football match.

In fact, the childish faces under the baseball caps had mannish stubble on them. The boys in the bus were not schoolchildren but Leopards and the bus had been specially hired for the day by the DEA. Although the policemen themselves did not know it — they had simply been told to dress in plain clothes and act the fool — they were about to attack the empire of one of Bolivia's largest drugs bosses, Carmelo 'Meco' Domínguez.

The aim of the operation, which the DEA had been planning for nine months, was to assault all parts of the organisation at once. There would be three strands to the operation: the Chapare, the Beni and Santa Cruz. In Santa Cruz it would destroy the Mafia's corporate headquarters by arresting key personnel, like lawyers, pilots and go-betweens, and would seize Meco's business assets, including Reginne's discotheque, a pharmacy and a Mitsubishi car showroom. In the Chapare, the bust would target Meco's paste-buying operations, run by a group called Los Huatos who operated out of Isinuta. In the Beni, a five-man commando team would raid a laboratory called Ascención de Guarayos, which reportedly made 12,000 to 15,000 kilograms of base a week, sold to the Cali and Medellín cartels in Colombia.

The DEA told as few people in the government as possible. So many operations had been mysteriously compromised at the last minute. You never quite knew in what private activities a politician was involved or what were his family connections. The DEA told only two men: General Lucio Añez, the head of the Special Force for the Fight Against Drug Trafficking, who was later to be ousted by Rico Toro, and Gonzálo Torrico, under-secretary for social defence in the Interior Ministry. The man most conspicuously kept in the dark was Capobianco. On the day the operation was carried out, he was 'coincidentally' out of the country.

In the long run, the DEA hoped the operation, if successful, would push the government into undertaking similar actions in the future. Once the Mafia had been destroyed, even those politicians with dubious connections would have little choice but to bring Domínguez to trial and stamp out the remaining tentacles of his network. Or so the DEA hoped.

The operation went exactly as in the textbooks. In the dead of night, the joint DEA/UMOPAR team landed their helicopter on the tiny airstrip hacked out of the Beni jungle at a place called Ascención de Guarayos. Two aircraft were parked on the strip. The team seized them, then proceeded to two ranches from where they knew aircraft flights into and out of laboratories in the Beni and Santa Cruz regions were controlled. At the first, called El Progreso, the team found a stash of arms. There was a 16-gauge shotgun with shells, a .22-calibre rifle and a .22-calibre revolver.

On their way back to the airstrip, the men found a cluster of tell-tale plastic barrels on the track which led them to a lab on the far side of a huge lake called Laguna las Aquiles, complete with kitchen, dormitories, drying and straining areas. The kitchen had seats for nine, and food for ten days. Nine sleeping bags were strewn on the bunks in the dormitory. The drying area, about 20 by 40 feet, had two drying tables and the usual propane tanks, heat lamps, water pumps and electric drills. Later the agents found another lab beside the Río Blanco with documents showing it was used by the paste-buying group, Los Huatos. The workers had escaped in canoes down the river when they heard the agents arrive.

Meanwhile in the Chapare, a few hundred miles south, for the previous four weeks the DEA and UMOPAR had been trying to smash the operations of Los Huatos. They had seized around 50 kilos of paste and base. On 23 September, four DEA agents and five Leopards had driven to a spot just behind Isinuta in the middle of the night. Leaving their vehicles with a UMOPAR security guard and a driver, they infiltrated into the jungle behind the town and set up a patrol base. Their aim was to catch members of Meco's organisation whom they knew were due to land on a strip north of the town to pick up around 450 kilos of base from Los Huatos. They also wanted to capture a particularly unsavoury character called Carmelo Rivera, nicknamed Rambo, who ran death squads for Meco.

Early on the morning of 24 September they were woken by machine-gun fire, a sign that the traffickers were about to buy. Their informant returned from town. 'The big buyers are there,' he said. 'There are 15 to 20 of them, all heavily armed. They're killing anyone who comes into town.' The agents sent the informant back to town. 'When they start buying we'll come in,' they told him.

The agents tuned into their high-frequency radios. They listened to the traffickers on one band and their driver, who was about to pick them up and drop them up-river, on another. They heard the paste dealers saying they were waiting for the aircraft to land. Then to their horror they realised the traffickers had heard their jeeps and were sending some thugs to destroy them.

'Fuck this,' said Tom South, a DEA medic. 'We've got to get those guys out or they'll be dead meat.'

The agents rushed to the vehicles, to find the driver and security guard and their jeeps under fire from 20 to 30 traffickers, armed to the teeth with M-16s, Uzis, and FNs. Behind them was a screaming mob of over 100 villagers. Having rescued the two Leopards, the agents came under fire themselves. A fierce gun-battle followed. The Americans radioed to Chimoré for help. One agent called Hawthorne Hope, nicknamed Archie, was hit in the ankle and the arm. 'I'm hit,' he gasped, as he jumped and fell to the ground. Dodging the bullets, which were flying in from 180 degrees, South yelled, 'I can't get you now. Crawl behind me and I'll pull you towards me.' The remaining agents meanwhile were emptying whole rounds on the trafficker who appeared to be leading the assault. 'If I see the motherfucker I'll kill him,' exclaimed one DEA agent as he fired from behind a rock. Finally they hit him and with relief watched his body float down the river. Archie crawled on all fours behind South.

Suddenly the traffickers regrouped and more thugs arrived as reinforcements. South, who had worked in some dodgy places in his time, including El Salvador, could not believe he was in peaceful Bolivia. The gunmen were smart too. They moved down from a twelve o'clock to a nine o'clock position to within 30 metres of the Americans. 'Rounds were flying by our heads and legs. It's amazing we didn't get shot. We were fighting for our lives,' recalls one agent. 'The whole town were out with their machetes. I thought they were going to chop us into bits.' South pushed Archie behind a tree stump and injected him with intravenous medication. He propped him upright and balanced his machine-gun in his hands. He could not give him pain-killers; Archie had to carry on fighting for his life.

Terrified the mob were going to move to a six o'clock position and close in on them, the agents retreated to a banana field. Finally they heard the buzz of two choppers which had arrived from Chimoré. They let off flares to indicate where they were. The traffickers turned their attention to the helicopters but were repelled after the crew fired their M-100 machine guns. Archie was rushed back to the base where he was attended by Special Forces medics. The other chopper took a team of agents south of Isinuta, where they set up a road-block and captured 16 of the traffickers. The two and a half hour battle was finally over. South alone had got through 235 rounds. It was a very close escape.

Meanwhile, agents were carrying out an assault on their third front, Santa Cruz. The bus-load of Leopards had managed to arrive in the city unnoticed and seized nine aircraft at Trompillo airport, seven of them Cessna 206s worth $60,000 each, plus a Cessna Caravan worth $725,000. A pilot and two aeroplane owners were arrested and two hangars seized. Meanwhile, other enforcement agents tackled the command and control of the Mafia's operation, seizing offices and documents, freezing bank accounts and apprehending businesses used as fronts for drugs money. Reginne's, valued at around $3 million, contained $100,000 in cash and crucial documents proving links with the Domínguez Mafia. At Domínguez's house, worth $230,000, the agents found more cash, radio systems and information about trafficking routes to Colombia, Mexico and the US.

Unlike previous operations, the Domínguez bust managed to catch the traffickers themselves. Finding his house surrounded by police, Domínguez gave himself up without a struggle. Lesser names, who ran the organisation's corporate headquarters in Santa Cruz and acted as intermediaries between Domínguez and the authorities he bought off, were also arrested.

The next stage was crucial. If a trafficker had been foolish or unlucky enough to get himself into a gaol cell, he would then pay the relevant legal authorities to let him out, or if that was not possible, to fiddle the evidence. This time the DEA were not going to let that happen. They hauled Meco and his men into a safe house for questioning, and filmed it on video camera. Accounts vary as to who carried out the interrogation. US officials say UMOPAR and the DEA both did it. Bolivian officials say the Americans insisted on doing it alone and kept the Bolivians out, despite the fact that US agents are barred from carrying out interrogations abroad. Meco and his men were sent to San Pedro.

The statements made by Meco and his intermediaries were a bombshell. They revealed a sophisticated network of payoffs which went higher than anyone had imagined. There were two men to whom Domínguez said he paid the biggest kickbacks: Capobianco and Carvajal.

Gelbard watched for the government's reaction. There was total silence.

As each day went by he was more and more surprised. There was only one explanation, he believed, and that was that some very key people were very uncomfortable. He rang Añez and Torrico. 'Why isn't your government taking any credit?' he asked. 'It doesn't look good.' The men responded non-committally. The most conspicuous silence was that of Capobianco, who had not said a word about the 'most successful drugs raid in Bolivian history'. 'That verified beliefs that the Domínguez Mafia was one of Capobianco's major sources of funding,' said one US diplomat.

Gelbard could not believe it. He knew it was vital to get the Bolivian government to claim credit for such a key drugs bust. That way it would be far harder for it to compromise any investigations that followed. Officials in Washington, like Bernard Aronson, Assistant Secretary for Inter-American Affairs, were instructed to make as much of it as possible in their dealings with Bolivian diplomats. 'We need to guard against the chance of compromise by Bolivian officials associated with the Meco organisation,' a La Paz-based US official told Washington. He went on:

> The down side is that the government of Bolivia may be reluctant now even to accept credit for the success. Some may (deliberately or otherwise) wind up turning success into a public relations problem on the principle of [cocaine] 'not invented here'. The government of Bolivia has always been loathe to associate itself closely with counter narcotics enforcement operations, which many prefer to treat as a favour Bolivia is doing for the United States.

This time, the official warned, it was vital to get the government to claim credit since 'leaders of the Meco organisation are identifying several Bolivian government officials by name as their corrupt interlocutors. Once second-tier arrests provide more documentation, we will need to get President Paz to clean up his government's act.'

Inside the Bolivian government a storm was brewing. Finally, ten days after Meco's arrest, Torrico made a bland statement to the press. Behind the scenes there was panic. According to US sources, Capobianco and Jaime Paz were very concerned about what Meco and his men had said, and were determined not to let a similar operation happen again. In particular, the sources claim, they were furious with General Añez, who had so clearly cooperated with the US in carrying out the raid. According to one Bolivian anti-narcotics official, government officials were livid because they had not been allowed into Meco's interrogation and had been barred even from seeing the video and documents. They had seen no proof that Meco had indeed said what the US said he had said. Old anti-imperialist sensitivities had been rudely reawakened: yet again the US had run the show without even consulting the top officials of the country in which they were operating.

For the next few months there was an uneasy calm. The US held its fire, believing the time was not yet ripe to reveal the names of high-ranking officials, including Capobianco, whom Meco and his men said were involved in the drugs trade. 'Capobianco's removal has been sought by us,' said one official at the time, 'but is not feasible because of the close personal and political relationship with Paz.' For the moment, the embassy would play along, using men like Torrico and Añez to get their way. The Bolivian government, meanwhile, was apparently closing ranks. A few months after the raid it summoned a key witness based in the Chapare to testify against Meco at a hearing in La Paz. The only snag was that it gave him only two hours' notice, and the Chapare was five hours away by plane at the very least, even assuming a commercial flight happened to be scheduled. Later the government appointed new policemen, many of whom the embassy believed were involved in drugs trafficking. As usual, the embassy objected, the matter was battled out and a few of the appointments were grudgingly rescinded.

The government allowed the odd drugs raid to be carried out, including a big clamp-down on the Red Zone in the Chapare, but none affected the big traffickers like the Meco raid had. 'They had to throw us bones here and there,' said a US official. 'They'd give us some dead labs, or some low-level traffickers. But none of the big shots.' One reason was that General Añez, the head of the Special Force for the Fight Against Drug Trafficking, whom the US believed was one of the few Bolivian authorities serious about fighting drugs, was in Brazil having two heart by-pass operations.

In April the following year, Meco escaped from San Pedro after he and a police guard left to 'visit a clinic'. After a nationwide man-hunt he was recaptured in Santa Cruz and returned to La Paz.

DOWN in the southern city of Cochabamba, far from the chill cobbled streets of the capital, a different drama was unfolding. Five years earlier, two unemployed lads from the mining city of Oruro, called Eddy and Nelson Arévalo, had appeared in town and put their $5,000 life savings into setting up a savings bank cum air taxi company called Firma Integral de Servicios Arévalo (Integral Company of Arévalo Services), or FINSA.

FINSA was not the first savings bank to have been set up in Cochabamba. There was already one called Multiactiva, which had been started during the García Meza regime and which had established a private university. What was new about FINSA was that it paid a phenomenal rate of interest, 7-8 per cent a month. *Cochabambinos* could not put their money into FINSA fast enough. FINSA FINSA FINSA was all anybody could talk about. Coca farmers who had been paid $2,000 in compensation for eradicating their hectare of coca ploughed the money into FINSA. Redundant miners from the Arévalos' home city of Oruro invested their 'relocation' money in it. Pensioners and housewives put their life savings into FINSA or mortgaged their homes to buy shares. Government ministers and police officers used FINSA to stash away the odd thousands of dollars they had quietly acquired. Rico Toro had either $80,000 or $250,000 in FINSA, depending on which report you believed. Carvajal allegedly had lots of money in it too. Even Bolivia's best-known Andean pop group, Las Kharkas, invested $600,000 in FINSA after winning $1.5 million in damages against a French company which filched one of its songs called *Llorando Se Fué* (He Left Crying) and passed it off as the *Lambada*. By early 1991 FINSA had an estimated 22,000 clients, compared with 6,000 a year earlier.

FINSA was particularly handy for one group of *cochabambinos*, the drug traffickers. The institution was ideal for laundering money. They could come in through the back door with suitcases of greenbacks. Officially, they would ask for a loan for an aeroplane or something and get their money back nice and clean. They put their properties, bought with recycled narco dollars and often operating at a loss, into the hands of FINSA. There was the city's glitzy night-club, Los Espejos (Mirrors), bought in 1988 by a former police major and alleged drugs trafficker, Bismarck Barrientos, and worth around $800,000. There were hotels, eight-floor apartment blocks of which only two floors were occupied, and a television station called Channel Nine.

Eddy and Nelson, now household names, became millionaires. They set up a radio taxi company whose telephone number, 2160, coincided with a famous 1985 decree allowing people (including druglords) to do what they wanted with their money with no questions asked. They bought an air taxi company, called Flash Tours, which was based at Cochabamba's airport and hired out small planes. They bought football teams in Cochabamba and in their home city of Oruro, and paid for a Brazilian coach to come and train them. In Cochabamba they bought the Cine Bustillo, virtually the only cinema in town that showed anything other than US westerns, but it soon closed. Eddy and Nelson moved into a $900,000 mansion in the city's exclusive Frutillar district, complete with football field, swimming pool and armed security guards. It even had its own private chapel which was used to bless the house when the brothers threw a huge house-warming party to which they invited all the local dignitaries.

But they did not spend all their money on themselves. Like many of the traffickers, the Arévalo brothers also had a paternalistic streak. They ordered clinics and schools to be built in the poor areas of town, just as the Colombian druglord Pablo Escobar had done in Medellín. In 1990 they paid for a Latin American congress for medical students and in 1991 they funded a Casa de Cultura, complete with theatre and library. Sometimes the brothers even graced the poor with their company. Seen as upright, God-fearing family men, they were hailed as heroes by their grateful beneficiaries. Notices went up around town saying *Gracias a FINSA*. The word went round that the brothers might stand in the December 1991 municipal elections.

Noting the Arévalos' success, others followed suit. Savings banks sprang up like mushrooms. The new entrepreneurs had three things in common with the Arévalo brothers: they were young, they came from outside

Cochabamba and they had no business or financial experience. Two banks were run by disc jockeys. Another, called Orcobol, was run by a former head of immigration. All paid between 5 and 7 per cent interest a month. The only thing savers had to do was to promise the money for three months and they would immediately get a month's interest in advance. Between them, the largest five, including FINSA, paid out around $1 million interest a month.

In their frenzy to get rich quick, few people bothered to ask questions. It did seem a bit odd to some people that FINSA could pay much higher interest than the ordinary banks. It was a bit puzzling, too, how FINSA could invest so much of its money in projects that offered no returns, such as half-built office blocks and football teams. But as long as demand kept up no-one really worried, since FINSA could pay interest with the new funds which were flooding in. Officials who could and should have examined the banks' finances were clearly not doing so.

Meanwhile, Wilson García, the quiet-spoken journalist on the local *Los Tiempos* newspaper, was doing what he believed to be his job: he was investigating FINSA and the other four main savings banks. His research, published in August 1990, opened a can of worms. With one exception, he discovered, the societies had refused to show their accounts when ordered to do so by a team of tax inspectors sent from La Paz in April. When the inspectors eventually gained access to the reluctant four, three weeks later, many of the relevant documents were 'missing'. The few accounts they could examine showed that the companies were totally unviable. None of them had records of their investments or feasibility studies to justify payment of around 70 per cent annual interest. None of the accounts balanced. FINSA, for example, had borrowed $50 million from its investors. Of that $10 million had been invested and $20 million spent paying interest to its borrowers. Where the other $20 million had gone was a mystery. It was the reverse with the smaller banks. Their investments were far larger than their assets. Either the books had been fiddled, or their owners had no clue about finance.

The most curious thing was that the societies deposited their savers' money, on which they were paying out 70 per cent a year, in ordinary banks which paid a maximum of 15 per cent. In other words, the societies were losing between 45 and 60 per cent of their liquidity every year. García also found that they were evading tax on a massive scale. 'Altogether the Treasury is losing around $103,000 a month,' he said in his report. 'What is odd is that neither the Inland Revenue nor the National Audit Office have taken measures to avoid this tax evasion.'

Investigative journalism, however, was not what the *cochabambinos* wanted. Investors were furious that García was slagging off the two respectable chaps who had given them so much money. Even angrier were the owners of the banks who had avoided adverse publicity. A day after the report appeared they held a meeting.

The next day, a sunny Tuesday morning, García walked from his house to the kiosk at the corner of his street to buy some cigarettes. Suddenly he felt a tap on his shoulder. He turned round, thinking it was a friend saying 'Hi'. As he did so, he felt a knife plunging into his stomach just below his heart. García could not breathe. 'You son of a bitch. Next time, you'll die,' García heard the man say before he blacked out. He thought he recognised the man, but he ran off before he had time to make sure.

The next thing García knew was that he was fighting for his life in the Belgian Medical Centre. Over the next three weeks he underwent five major operations. He would have stayed longer, but his treatment had already cost him $10,000 and he knew that he would not get any help from the authorities.

Convalescing at home, García received a string of threatening phone calls. 'If you investigate the incident,' one voice said, 'it will be worse next time.' García knew he was not joking. He did not go anywhere without a weapon and a UMOPAR bodyguard. But the police guard was reluctant to protect García, particularly as he was missing out on the 'bonuses' that his colleagues were getting. García also found it tiresome having his every movement watched with a hawk's eye. He decided the bodyguard was probably more of a liability than a protection and he got rid of him. García knew that the local authorities were so corrupt that there was nowhere he could turn for justice. He was totally alone.

ON 4 February 1991, the DEA's aircraft experts and a group of Leopards were carrying out routine checks on the small aeroplanes that used Cochabamba's airport. They spotted a couple parked on the far side of the tarmac and the tail number of one of these matched that of a single-engine plane they had seen taking off from the Chapare a few weeks earlier. They suspected they might belong to Bismarck Barrientos. They consulted General Añez, head of the Special Force, who ordered the DEA's chemist to carry out a 'carpet test'. This entails sweeping the floors of a plane with a special hoover which tests for traces of cocaine. The result was positive.

They fed the tail numbers into the computer to find out to whom they belonged. To their amazement, the computer came up with the Arévalos.

Confusion followed as the DEA tussled with the Bolivian authorities to bring the owners of the planes to justice. Every move the US and Añez made was blocked by counter orders from above. Twelve people were arrested but, apart from three pilots, all were released. By the time Añez had ordered the brothers' arrest, they had disappeared, along with police evidence on the case. While things were being sorted out the government froze FINSA's assets.

A few days after the seizure, Añez got a call from Capobianco. 'It's easy for you to carry out a *narco* test,' Capobianco warned him. 'But it creates one hell of a lot of problems for the government.' Añez said nothing, but wondered what a head of the Special Force was supposed to do if it was not tracing cocaine.

In Cochabamba, meanwhile, there was furore. The FINSA bubble had finally burst, leaving thousands of ordinary *cochabambinos* destitute. The Las Kharkas pop group smarted as the irony of the words of the song (*He Left Crying*) which had brought it the funds to invest in FINSA became apparent. People rushed to pull out their savings, but it was too late: the estimated $30 million that FINSA owed had disappeared into thin air. Some went on hunger strike to demand back their savings. Others thronged into Cochabamba's main square and staged marches to protest against what they dubbed the *estafa del siglo* (swindle of the century). Some held a mass to celebrate the anniversary of FINSA's founding and to protest the Arévalos' innocence. They were angry with Eddy and Nelson, but they were even more irate with the authorities who had interfered and unfairly accused the young men of being involved in drugs trafficking. The worst culprits, they muttered, were the DEA, the government and meddling journalists like Wilson García.

La Paz, meanwhile, was in political turmoil. The government was furious with General Añez, who had not only smashed the Meco Mafia but had now destroyed FINSA as well. At 6.00 p.m. on 4 March Añez received a phone call at his office from Capobianco telling him that he had better step down. He gave no reason. Añez went straight to the Interior Ministry where he found a resignation letter waiting for him to sign which said he was leaving on 'health grounds'. Añez signed it at 7.45 p.m. A mere 30 seconds later Rico Toro was appointed in his place.

Rico Toro lost no time. Within 24 hours of his inauguration he had declared that the Arévalo brothers had nothing to do with drugs trafficking and had sent a letter to this effect to Torrico. In a secret deal he agreed that Eddy, Nelson and the pilots would be released 'under guarantee' on the grounds that there was insufficient proof to detain them. In exchange, government and police officials, including Rico Toro himself, would get their money back. One police commander had already taken the matter into his own hands. He had kidnapped the brothers as they had tried to escape into Brazil and refused to release them until they paid him back the $280,000 he had put into FINSA.

This time Wilson García did not investigate. On the day the planes were seized he sent an anodyne report to a newspaper in La Paz but did nothing for *Los Tiempos*. But even that annoyed somebody. At 3.00 a.m. the next morning the telephone rang in his home. García's mother answered. 'Your time has come,' said the voice. From then on, terrified for his life, García only ventured out to go to work. Death threats arrived daily, traumatising García's family. His mother could no longer sleep. His two brothers sought psychiatric help.

ON A HUMID Sunday afternoon two weeks later there was a festive atmosphere in Cochabamba's central square, where crowds had thronged and seemed to be waiting for something to happen. A brass band of chubby-faced Indians was playing, punctuated every now and then by bursts of gunfire. Under the palm trees outside the cathedral, women were busy preparing garlands of white orchids.

Tourists staying in the city imagined it must be yet another fiesta to celebrate yet another national holiday. Looking closer, however, they noticed that the banners being waved were not the usual red, green and yellow Bolivian flags, but referred to FINSA. '*Los pobres con FINSA, los ricos con los bancos ineficientes*' (The poor with FINSA, the rich with the inefficient banks) read one, daubed in red paint on an old white sheet. 'Cochabamba we want you free, without the DEA. FINSA worked for the poor. We don't want people who live off the sweat of the people,' read another. 'We want our aeroplanes,' said another. Outside the town hall, policemen fidgeted nervously.

Suddenly the band struck up and the crowd began to cheer. 'It's them,' exclaimed one old man, who seemed oblivious of being nearly crushed to death by the heaving mob. On the platform beneath the condor-topped independence column in the centre of the square appeared the two Arévalo brothers and a diminutive woman who was weeping with emotion, the *mamá*. The boys, festooned with garlands of white orchids like bride-grooms, stared open mouthed, lapping up the applause. For the masses, it was a sacred moment. One tourist who tried to take a snap was jeered angrily. 'This isn't the kind of thing you take photographs of,' said one middle-aged woman, presumably one of the thousands of savers who believed they were now about to get their money back. 'It's serious.'

The crowd hushed as the boys began to speak. Eddy began.

> FINSA is not a company which sprang up overnight. We have helped the poor, we have carried out humanitarian acts, without ever expecting reward. *Compañeros*, I am a father, I have children, how would I do anything that hurt society?... [Cheers and shouts, then hush again.]... We have helped sport, culture, all for the good of society. We are your humble servants. Our struggle will not end until our company is working again.

The crowd cheered again. Nelson took over.

I pay homage to all you noble workers, men and women, who are on hunger strike. Let us show the government how this company works, let us show that sham of a DEA which wanted to destroy FINSA, which wanted to destroy thousands of poor people. Help me declare that FINSA united will never be destroyed. Long live FINSA, long live Bolivia.

Riding the wave of hysteria, the crowd joined in. 'Long live FINSA.'

The speeches over, the two heroes were paraded, shoulder-high, around the square. They finished up at the town hall where a group of policemen ushered them in as deferentially as if they had been the mayor. Night was falling and the crowd began to drift off home, drunk with emotion. A small group of women, though, remained. They had constructed an altar on the back of their pick-up truck in front of the cathedral and adorned it with orchids and incense. In the silence of the night, weeping women prayed and chanted to thank God for a truly momentous day.

Six months later, Nelson was dead.

The police found his body slumped over the front seat of his sky-blue Suzuki just after breakfast on 30 September after a child spotted blood trickling to the ground from the landcruiser's front door. A bullet had blasted through his head just above his right ear and emerged above his left. On the back seat was an empty black briefcase. In a strange coincidence, that same day Nelson had been due to pay back some of the estimated $50,000 he owed to around 20,000 people. Forensic experts estimated the body had been dead for three to four hours.

Nelson had spent the day before he died with his family. In the evening he had left his mansion on the outskirts of town on a mystery assignment after telling his bodyguards to go to bed. He had taken with him a briefcase, which Nelson's brother Eddy later claimed Nelson had been about to fill with the money which he was to pick up from an intermediary so that he could pay it out to depositors the following day. Cochabambinos living in the neighbourhood swore they had not heard a single shot.

When the police found him, Nelson's body was bent double and so rigid they could not get him out of the car. So they took both the body and the car to the morgue for an autopsy. The body was still clad in the dapper white trousers, striped shirt and coffee-coloured jacket Nelson had put on for his secret rendezvous.

The news flew round the city. Weeping women gathered at the spot where Nelson had died and followed him to the morgue. Later they trailed the corpse to the discotheque *Reflejos* where a long wake began. The next day the body was taken to the central square where Nelson had received a hero's welcome in March so that admirers could pay homage to him before a funeral mass was held in the cathedral. They praised his 'honourable' character and the work he had done for the poor.

Savers declared a 'state of emergency' and congregated in thousands at the square. Others rapped on the doors of FINSA to enquire how Nelson had died. They were sure the blame lay with the government, who they claimed had tried to destroy FINSA by linking it with drug trafficking. They demanded FINSA be instantly legalised and the drug trafficking charges dropped.

Every aspect of FINSA had been shrouded in mystery, but the death of its 33-year-old president was surely the greatest riddle of them all. Nelson had so many enemies it was hard to guess which one might have been responsible. Was it a disgruntled depositor who wanted his or her money back? Or was it the agent of some government official who had made some kind of deal with Nelson which had now gone wrong? Had an intermediary, charged with handing over a large sum of money to Nelson, instead decided to kill him and run off with the cash? Or, knowing that he could not avoid paying back his investors any longer, had Nelson decided to take his own life?

None of the evidence the investigators found quite pieced together and much was contradictory. Some of the most interesting came from a woman called Liliana Fatima Benigna Adriazoza who had worked as Nelson's secretary since May 1989 and then became his lover. She pointed the finger at a shadowy organisation called 'Group X', presumed to represent FINSA investors, which she claimed had pursued Nelson and threatened him with 'little presents and surprises'. Once, she alleged, the group had broken into Nelson's office and left a note threatening to blow it up.

Eddy backed up Liliana's claim by producing a photocopy of a letter, dated 7 August, allegedly signed by Group X. 'We will look after everything, don't interfere because your life is in danger,' the letter continued. 'You are no longer needed in Bolivia, so stop fucking us around and leave the solution to this mess in our hands. Sleep calmly as we are looking after you and your family carefully.'

Another possibility, according to Liliana, was that Nelson had taken his own life. She said Nelson had told her on numerous occasions that he wanted to kill himself because he knew he could never pay back his depositors. 'Nelson told me he was ruined, lost in a blind alley,' she told investigators. During the harrowing last six months of his life, Nelson had lived a life of perpetual terror, she said.

Other evidence pointed the finger at the men who were supposed to protect Nelson, his bodyguards. Knowing Nelson was about to receive a large sum of money, they could have killed him and run off with it. They could have acted on their own behalf, or as agents of someone else. Alternatively, Nelson could have ordered them to kill him. This theory was backed up by the discovery of a note in which Nelson allegedly offered a $50,000 reward for carrying out the deed.

One of the most interesting threads of the mystery, however, involved a man called Jaime Escobar, one of Bolivia's top banking regulatory officials who had been Finance Minister in the 1960s. According to Eddy, Escobar had made a deal with Nelson under which he had legalised FINSA in return for a very large 'incentive' from Nelson. Eddy claimed the 'incentive' amounted to $3 million.

A month and a half before Nelson's death, a telex had been sent from La Paz to Cochabamba signed by 'your friend of always, Jaime' on which Nelson had allegedly scribbled 'Telex received from Dr Escobar, chief inspector of banks'. In the communication Escobar reportedly asked Nelson to be patient and not to bother him by phone. 'Little brother', he concluded, 'be patient, we will make your dream of having your own bank come true.'

Something then seems to have gone wrong. Two weeks before his death Nelson allegedly sent a letter to Escobar demanding that Escobar return the $3 million. Nelson was apparently to use the money to pay back some of his investors and to buy a front company behind which FINSA could function again. It was not clear when or how Escobar was to hand over the money. Eddy's theory was that an agent of Escobar's had killed Nelson as a way of avoiding paying back the $3 million.

Escobar, of course, denied that any money had exchanged hands between him and Nelson, although he did admit that Nelson had sought a meeting with him in La Paz on 25 September. But he said it had never happened because Nelson's flight from Cochabamba had been cancelled because of a bomb scare.

The mystery surrounding Escobar deepened still further with the discovery of a cassette — hauntingly similar to the narco-video involving Roberto Suarez and his ADN cronies — which allegedly carried a conversation between Escobar's daughter, Maria Eugenia, Nelson, and an MNR deputy called Franklin Anaya, supposedly acting as Nelson's 'adviser'. According to police statements, Nelson is heard to offer a bribe to the woman's father in return for the legalisation of FINSA and the closure of several rival savings banks. The amount mentioned on the tape is $300,000 — well short of the $3 million alleged by Eddy. The money would be distributed among government functionaries and put into party coffers. Maria Eugenia allegedly promises to convince her father to cooperate. At one point she even telephones him. 'OK,' Nelson concludes at the end. 'Everything is arranged.' The cassette was allegedly released in La Paz by the head of FINSA's investors, a man called Jaime Gutiérrez, but its authenticity will probably never be proved. Anaya denied the voice on the tape was his, although he admitted he had had political links with Nelson because both had worked in the youth branch of the MNR.

The truth about how Nelson died will probably never be known.

CORRUPTION has always been an obstacle to the carrying out of campaigns against the cocaine trade. This is hardly surprising, given the huge quantities of money mobilised by the traffickers, and the relative poverty of the people they pay off, whether politicians, policemen or judges. Politicians are paid miserable salaries by Western standards, and can only survive if they have extra sources of funding. 'Many deputies are paid so badly they don't want to do the job any more,' says Lauro Ocampo, an MIR deputy, who says his colleagues earn a maximum of $1,000 a month. 'That's nothing when you consider that rent on a house is $400. Then there are school fees for the children, and so on.'

Not everyone in the government gets kickbacks. To pay off everyone would not make financial sense for the traffickers. Instead, they buy people in key positions, like the interior and defence ministers, the head of customs, the person responsible for giving licences for the import of chemicals, and so on. But because corruption has long been a way of life in Bolivia and is so widespread, few politicians feel bought. 'If the drug industry didn't pay off government officials, it would be the only industry in Bolivia that didn't,' says a US official. 'It's a business like any other.' A Bolivian politician agrees, 'Protection money doesn't dirty you, you don't handle the stuff, you just say when there's going to be a strike and money appears in your account.'

Politicians rely on the drug barons as a source of funds for their parties and increasingly costly election campaigns. Usually traffickers give to all three parties as an insurance policy. 'Every trafficker with the savvy to come in from the rain pays off the political parties,' says one US official. According to Captain Sempértegui, who investigated the narco-video scandal, Roberto Suárez promised to contribute $200,000 to the ADN's 1989 election campaign. US sources estimate the 1993 election campaign will cost the ruling MIR party between $15 and $20 million. Not surprisingly, attempts to establish a federal election commission, which would examine each party's finances, have been stillborn.

Bolivia is also a tiny country in terms of population. With barely seven million people, among the middle and upper classes everybody knows and is related to everybody else. Family ties dominate politics. They also play an important role when it comes to fighting drugs trafficking, since virtually every politician has some kind of blood link, albeit distant, with a cocaine trafficker. The trafficker tends to be dismissed as a 'black sheep' rather than a criminal. With the family still the sacred centre of every Bolivian's life, touching a relative would be unthinkable. On the other hand, it should be added that there are politicians who would shun contact with a trafficker, at least publicly. Some ask the DEA to identify traffickers and then make sure they have nothing to do with them. A number have got *narcos* expelled from exclusive clubs.

As the events of 1990 and 1991 showed, drug corruption influences government decisions when it comes to fighting, or not fighting, cocaine. But other considerations are equally important.

One is the crucial role that cocaine plays in the national economy. This makes politicians adopt a pragmatic as opposed to a moral stance to the drugs problem. Being illegal, there are no exact figures on its contribution to Bolivia's economy. Estimates vary from $300 to $700 million, or between 6 and 12 per cent of its GNP.[3] All economists agree that cocaine is by far the country's largest export (equivalent to around 90 per cent of legal exports), and a crucial source of foreign exchange. Cocaine money plays a key role in stabilising the exchange rate and keeping inflation low. The money is ploughed into the national economy under a 'no questions asked' decree passed by President Paz Estenssoro in 1985. Without the influx of coca dollars Bolivia would have found it extremely difficult to stick to its economic stabilisation plan, introduced by Estenssoro and still in place today, hailed by the West as a success of neo-liberal economic policies. Lacking the violence of the cocaine trade in Colombia, Bolivia's drugs trade has not had a significant enough effect on tourism and foreign investment to make politicians adopt a negative view.

The industry is also one of the most important providers of jobs and income in a country with around 15 per cent official unemployment. About 5 per cent of Bolivia's seven million population work directly in the drugs trade, and a further 15 per cent if one includes all the construction workers, lawyers, cooks, bankers and others in legal jobs who survive by selling services to the industry. The impact of eliminating the coca industry would be equivalent to laying off some tens of millions of people in the US.

In the long term, politicians recognise the disadvantages of cocaine, such as the loss of tax revenue, the erosion of law and order, and the 'Dutch disease' effect, whereby the cocaine industry sucks labour and skills out of other sectors. The strong currency which results from cocaine money hurts exports, and Bolivia's dependence on cocaine damages its relations with international financial institutions like the IMF and World Bank. Deforestation, water pollution and increasing drugs addiction are also seen as serious problems. Politicians recognise that the cocaine boom will not last for ever. But they believe they can only be expected to dismantle the cocaine economy if a viable alternative can be installed in its place. This thinking, together with the fear of a peasant backlash, lies behind Jaime Paz's *Coca por Desarrollo* (Coca for Development) thesis, whereby Bolivia pledges to destroy its coca fields in exchange for real national development.

In the short term, though, with so many people's livelihoods dependent on cocaine, the social and political costs of eliminating the industry would be devastating. The coca growers are a numerous, well organised and powerful group. Few politicians want to push them too far for fear of sparking off a Peruvian-style insurgency. As Herber Muller, former director of Bolivia's Central Bank, put it, 'Cocaine is like a cushion that is preventing social explosion.' Politicians know that repressive anti-drugs policies will not win them votes. The only ones that will are ones that fill people's stomachs, like those promoting alternative development. As one US official admitted, 'A politician has no incentive to fight cocaine as it doesn't win him a single vote. The only people who want him to do anything are those at the US embassy. Politicians are afraid of disturbing the status quo in case it upsets their fragile democracy. They feel it's not worth their while.'

Politicians are also unwilling to upset the cocaine traffickers and, because of their lack of violence, have little incentive to do so. Despite fears that they might (or have) become so powerful that they could effectively control Bolivia, most politicians believe that the current *modus vivendi* is preferable to outright confrontation of the kind that occurred in Colombia. 'Let's not tread on the rattlesnake', is the view of most members of the present government, according to one opposition politician. 'Politicians say don't let's get too tough on them and they'll not get tough on us. They want to establish a peaceful coexistence with the *narcos* while doing the minimum to keep the Americans off their backs.' Some US officials viewed the government's 1991 decree, promising reduced gaol terms and no extradition if traffickers gave themselves up within 120 days, in this light. Like Colombia, Bolivia was able to achieve three things: it was seen to be taking moves to solve the narcotics problem peacefully; by banning extradition it defended national pride and put the US embassy in its place; and it kept the traffickers happy by promising them what were likely to be lenient prison sentences in Bolivia.

Underlying politicians' attitudes is the belief that cocaine is a *gringo* problem which should be tackled by *gringos*. It is the US craving for cocaine that has created the industry, they argue. Bolivia simply supplies the raw materials for which there is demand, in the same way as it used to supply the world with silver and tin. The fact that cocaine is illegal makes no difference. As a former tin-mine owner remarked, 'We are used to seeing our raw materials exported. Our exports have always been put to good and bad use.' In other words, if *gringos* want to snort cocaine that is their problem, not Bolivia's. As with other commodities, cocaine has not brought great wealth to Bolivia. The big profits have gone into the pockets of Colombian and US dealers. In Bolivia, although the industry has made a handful of entrepreneurs very rich, overall it has left the country as dirt-poor as it was before.

As a result Bolivian politicians are reluctant to bear the social, economic and human costs of fighting what they see as North America's war (supposing they were able to) and resent being beaten with Uncle Sam's 'big stick'. By portraying Bolivia as the 'source' of the drugs problem, the US effectively transfers the costs of the war to Bolivia, forcing it to carry out repressive anti-drugs measures it knows would be a liability if carried out at home in the US. Imagine the outcry, for example, if the US authorities destroyed their farmers' crops by spraying them with herbicides from the air, or if US citizens continually had their houses searched and robbed by police.

While forcing Bolivia to make drugs its top priority, the US seems to be incapable or unwilling to control its marijuana growers in California, or the banks that launder billions of narco dollars, as shown by the scandal involving the Bank of Credit and Commerce International in 1991. The resentment felt by South Americans was illustrated by Francisco Bernal, former head of Colombia's Narcotics Bureau within the office of the Attorney General, who said in 1988: 'We're being left to fight this war alone. We're supplying the dead, the country is being destabilised, and what help are we getting?' In contrast to US policy makers who characterise drugs as a threat to national security, Bolivians see repressive anti-drug measures, particularly using the military, as a far greater threat.

Like it or not, cocaine dominates and will continue to dominate relations between Bolivia and the US. Issues on which many Bolivians would prefer to focus, like poverty, debt and economic crisis, pale into insignificance beside drugs. On the positive side, though, drugs have brought Bolivia economic aid on a scale it will never again receive. 'Bolivia is a marginal country of no strategic importance to the US,' says MIR deputy Lauro Ocampo. 'Now drugs have turned us into a high priority. Drugs is our key negotiating card. Without drugs we would not have won half the economic aid we now get.' Bolivia is keen to lessen this dependence by building up links with Japan and Europe.

There are other limitations on Bolivia's willingness to wage an all-out war on drugs: the fact that other issues like economic crisis and political instability are seen as priorities; the weakness and corruption of institutions like the judiciary and the police force which politicians can do little to combat; and plain poverty, which means the country lacks the resources to fund anti-drugs programmes or to pay decent wages to those involved in fighting drugs; and, above all, its belief that US policy puts undue emphasis on short-term military-style solutions at the expense of long-term economic ones. Gradually though, Bolivians may be changing their attitudes, largely because addiction in Bolivia is growing at a devastating rate. While the issue of drugs was conspicuously absent from the 1989 election campaign, opinion polls indicate it will feature prominently in the 1993 campaign, although it will still undoubtedly lag behind issues like unemployment and political stability.

Bolivia's politicians face a no-win situation. International pressure is forcing them to cut off their life-support machine, which could in turn overturn the country's fragile democracy and economy. Failure to combat cocaine, on the other hand, would cut off another lifeline, US economic aid, and eat away further at the country's moral core, fostering an atmosphere of cynicism and virtual anarchy. It is a choice most politicians do not want to face.

9

Afterword

Our remedies often in ourselves do lie
Which we ascribe to heaven

Shakespeare: 'All's Well That Ends Well'

IN February 1992, President Bush met five Latin American presidents in San Antonio, Texas, for a two-day summit to discuss progress in fighting the drug menace. Two-and-a-half years after Bush had first announced his strategy, the assembled leaders seemed to have good reason to congratulate themselves. Drug seizures were up world-wide, demand for coke in the US was down, the ringleaders of Colombia's Medellín cartel were either dead or behind bars, and cocaine export routes had been disrupted.

But behind the official smiles was a bleaker reality. The presence of leaders of five Latin American countries — not just Colombia, Peru and Bolivia, but Ecuador and Mexico too — underlined the fact that coke traffickers, hounded in Colombia, have expanded geographically to countries like Bolivia, Mexico and Venezuela. Although coke seizures have increased, the overall flow from the region has soared to record levels. Efforts to stem the flood have been, as one US critic put it, 'like standing under a waterfall with a bucket.'

As things are, with its vast resources, the chances of Cocaine Inc. being forced to the wall and going bust are remote indeed. Like any business, it responds to changing market conditions by altering management and location. High profile anti-drug campaigns, changes in fashions or a surplus in supplies prompt it to switch consumer markets. Having saturated the US market, the coke barons are exporting instead to Europe and Japan, where consumers will pay at least three times the US price and where demand is rising. Prospects for expansion are excellent, especially in the countries of Eastern Europe and the former Soviet Union, whose populations are eager to savour what they see as the fruits of capitalism after decades of communist rule.

Finding employees to run the gauntlet of smuggling cocaine supplies across international borders, however risky, will never be difficult given the enormous sums the druglords can afford to pay. Cocaine Inc's multi-billion-dollar wealth will always enable it to corrupt the highest of officials in producer, transit and consumer countries.

Poverty and deprivation are prime reasons why South American peasants grow coca and why inhabitants of inner-city ghettoes of the US and Europe consume cocaine. Solving these problems, say some experts, is the key to eradicating the cocaine menace. Such a scenario, however, is pitifully remote, particularly at a time when the world is in deep recession. In fact, most South Americans are getting not richer but poorer as their governments wrestle with huge debt burdens and falling commodity prices. For many peasant farmers, coca is the only escape from grinding poverty. Corruption — to a large extent rooted in poverty and underdevelopment — is so endemic in South American societies that it will not be eradicated in the near future. On the streets of London and New York, too, recession has brought unemployment and misery on an unprecedented scale. In many cases, this has pushed people towards cocaine, a habit they are unlikely to kick until the underlying causes have been tackled.

Experts have offered a range of possible measures which could help tackle the cocaine problem. One is for Western countries to provide coca-producing countries with large injections of aid and expertise which would enable them to wean their economies off cocaine and compensate for the loss of a highly profitable industry. For this to work, Western countries would at the same time need to open their markets to alternative exports from coca-producing countries, ease trade barriers and take steps to alleviate broader economic problems in South American countries, like debt and economic stagnation. (Unfortunately, in Texas President Bush was unable to offer any new aid to the Andean presidents, arguing there was no money left in the recession-hit pot.)

Another suggestion is for 'debt for drugs' swaps, under which countries like the US would forgive the interest of Andean nations' debts in exchange for successful anti-narcotics programmes. (Though what would constitute 'successful' would be a likely source of debate.) Experts have also called for tighter controls on the production and transport of precursor chemicals and on the laundering of drug money. International agreements drawn up to control both these activities have had some success. But product controls can always be evaded and national or international laws are effectively powerless when it comes to monitoring the use and transport of chemicals in many of South America's vast expanses of jungle.

Other measures suggested by experts include improvements in Andean judicial, prison and political institutions to weaken the hold of the traffickers and ensure they are properly tried; improved education and prevention in consumer countries to help cut demand; and decriminalisation or legalisation of drugs which, proponents argue, would lead to a collapse in their price. This last option, which would treat drugs as a public health, rather than a criminal, problem, has many factors in its favour but is unlikely ever to be adopted given that law-makers in countries like the US consider the idea of legalising drug use morally repugnant or contrary to current policy.

Most of these measures have been tried to some extent. No single measure is sufficient on its own, and the policies will only be workable if Western and South American countries coordinate their actions — difficult given their differing viewpoints. Until now, lack of such coordination, of funds and of political will, have meant that measures like the ones suggested above have been stillborn. Western countries often appear to support a policy but then fail to provide the finance which would enable it to work.

Even clearer are the ways in which the cocaine menace should *not* be tackled. First, although law enforcement targeted at large-scale traffickers has a role to play in any anti-drugs strategy, guns and soldiers will never get rid of cocaine. They tackle the symptoms but do little to cure the causes. In Bolivia, with its history of coups, using the military will create far worse problems than those it is supposed to solve. Foreign countries that force Andean nations to use troops — which would be unacceptable at home — are not only being hypocritical but risk undermining the hard-won democracies they claim to support. Second, it is unrealistic to view coca in moralistic terms: peasants who grow coca do not do so because they are criminals, but because they have to survive. To repeat the words of the US official in Chapter Two, 'They are not addicted to coca, they are addicted to eating.' Moral reprobation is only in order when dealing with large-scale cocaine barons and their ruthless methods. Third, undue attention should not be placed on supplier countries. Equal — some say greater — attention should be paid to tackling demand, without which no-one would grow coca in the first place.

Ultimately, the problem, and the solution, lies in ourselves. Rather than just tackling the symptoms — labs, traffickers and paste pits — are we willing to eradicate the causes which prompt coca farmers to grow coca, or people in the West to consume cocaine and crack? Until we are, the 'war' will never be won.

Notes and References

Chapter 1

1. Senate judiciary committee report, 11 May 1990.

2. 'Cocaine: middle-class high,' *Time Magazine*, 6 July 1981.

3. 'Washington today, London by 1991?' *Sunday Times Magazine*, 1 April 1989.

4. 'Crack, bane of inner city is now gripping suburbs,' *New York Times*, 10 January 1990.

5. Ibid.

6. *Overview of Selected Drug Trends*, National Institute on Drug Abuse, January 1990.

7. J. Inciardi, 'Beyond cocaine: basuco, crack and other coca products,' *Contemporary Drug Problems*, 1988.

8. R. H. Schwartz, N. G. Hoffman and M. Luxemburg, 'Adolescents who smoke "crack": patterns and consequences of use,' *American Journal of Diseases of Children*, 1989.

9. 'Crisis in US spawns theories but no facts,' *Wall Street Journal*, 17 September 1989.

10. Ibid.

11. Quoted by C. Youngers and P. Andreas, 'US policy and the Andean cocaine industry,' *World Policy Journal*, Summer 1989.

12. 'Getting tough on cocaine,' *Newsweek*, 28 November 1988.

13. 'Kill the coca at its roots,' *Los Angeles Times*, 26 April 1990.

14. 'Guns, drugs and politics,' *Newsweek*, 28 July 1986.

15. C. Youngers and P. Andreas, 'US drug policy and the Andean cocaine industry,' *World Policy Journal*, Summer 1989.

16. DOS Inspector General Report, January 1990.

17. 'Cooperation among agencies deemed vital as president prepares for address,' *New York Times*, 5 September 1989.

18. 'The drug warrior,' *Newsweek*, 10 April 1989.

19. Ibid.

20. 'Bennett to resign as chief of US anti-drug effort,' *New York Times*, 7 November 1990.

21. A. Messing Junior and A. Hazlewood, *The US drug control policy and international operations*, June 1990.

22. Quoted in 'Proposal is a marked shift from border interdiction,' *Washington Post*, 27 May 1988.

23. 'Kill the coca at its roots,' *Los Angeles Times*, 26 April 1990.

24. The idea was not new. During the height of the heroine epidemic of the early 1970s, for example, President Nixon was excited by reports that a biologically engineered worm could be developed that would eat opium poppies. Nixon ordered a crash $2 million programme to develop the worm at Agriculture Department laboratories in Mississippi, according to *Agency of Fear* by Edward Epstein. But the project ran aground when alarmed State Department officials warned that if the worms were let loose on the illicit poppy fields of Afghanistan and Turkey they might soon migrate to the licit poppy fields of the Soviet Union, causing an international incident.

25. 'US considering plan to defoliate coca crops in Peru and Bolivia,' *Washington Post*, 11 March 1990.

26. Ibid.

27. Congressional Research Service, *Combating international drug cartels: issues for US policy*, Washington DC, September 1987.

28. Committee on Government Operations, *United States anti-narcotics activities in the Andean region*, November 1990.

29. 'Our troops shouldn't be drug cops,' *Washington Post*, 22 May 1988.

30. 'It is a matter of national security: use every weapon,' *Baltimore Sun*, 18 May 1988.

31. Statement by Melvyn Levitsky before Subcommittees on Western Hemisphere Affairs and Terrorism, Narcotics and International Operations Committee on Foreign Relations, US Senate, 28 June 1990.

Chapter 2

1. United Nations Development Programme, *Human development report 1991*, Oxford University Press.

2. The first is the figure given by the US State Department, the second by the Bolivian government.

3. US State Department figure.

4. 'Cocaine makers give the Amazon a toxic overdose,' *Sunday Times*, 30 December 1990.

5. J. Hemming, *The conquest of the Incas*, Penguin, 1983.

6. 'Guns, drugs and politics,' *Newsweek*, 29 July 1986.

7. US Senate Judiciary Committee and the International Narcotics Control Caucus, *The president's drug strategy: one year later*, September 1990.

8. Development Alternatives Inc, *Regional planning and strategy analysis for the Chapare Development Project*, July 1990.

9. Ibid.

Chapter 3

1. M. Levine, *Deep Cover*, Delacorte Press, 1990.

2. 'Bolivia cocaine output soars,' *Los Angeles Times*, 20 July 1990.

3. General Pereda seized power in a military coup in July 1978, but was ousted in November the same year.

4. Oral interrogatory, Lucerne, 27 January 1982.

5. M. Linklater *et al.*, *The Fourth Reich: Klaus Barbie and the neo-Fascist connection*, Hodder & Stoughton, 1984.

6. Ibid.

7. Information on the sting based on testimony from US vs Alfredo Gutiérrez, Roberto Suárez senior and junior, Marcelo Ibáñez, Renato Roca Suárez, 30 June 1980; affidavit of Richard Fiano; report of investigation by DEA undercover agent José Hinojosa, 16 June 1980.

8. M. Levine, *Deep Cover*, Delacorte Press, 1990.

9. B. Freemantle, *The Fix*, Tom Doherty Associates, 1985.

10. Oral interrogatory, Lucerne, 27 January 1982.

11. US vs Alfredo Gutiérrez, Roberto Suárez senior and junior, Marcelo Ibáñez, Renato Roca Suárez, 30 June 1980.

Chapter 4

1. US Congressional Committee on Government Operations, *Stopping the flood of cocaine with Operation Snowcap: is it working?* 14 August 1990.

Chapter 5

1. Historians disagree over the number of coups Bolivia has had. This is the figure most often quoted.

2. M. Linklater *et al.*, *The Fourth Reich*, Hodder & Stoughton, 1984.

3. Ibid.

4.   B. Freemantle, *The Fix*, Tom Doherty Associates, 1985.

5.   E. Shannon, *Desperados*, Viking Penguin, 1988.

6.   Latin American Weekly Report, 22 August 1980.

7.   M. Linklater *et al.*, *The Fourth Reich*, Hodder & Stoughton, 1984.

8.   Ibid.

9.   Ibid.

10.   Figure quoted in 'Bond denied for former interior chief,' *Miami Herald*, 4 January 1990.

11.   Latin American Weekly Report, 27 February 1981.

12.   Interview with Lupe Andrade, *Ultima Hora*, 15 April 1991.

13.   Ibid.

14.   'Techo de Paja y sus amigos de uniforme,' *Facetas de Los Tiempos*, 17 January 1988.

15.   Quoted in 'Bolivia resists drug role for army,' *Christian Science Monitor*, 7 May 1990.

16.   Informe R No 215, April 1991.

17.   Prepared statement of Melvyn Levitsky, assistant secretary of state for International Narcotics Matters before the Subcommittees on Western Hemisphere Affairs and Terrorism, Narcotics and International Operations, Committee on Foreign Relations, US Senate, June 28 1990.

18.   Quoted in US Congressional Committee on Government Operations report, *Stopping the flood of cocaine with Operation Snowcap: is it working?* 14 August 1990.

Chapter 6

1.   'Rough justice in Bolivia', *Independent Magazine*, 16 December 1989.

Chapter 7

1.   Jaime is not his real name. Real names of all temporary agents have been changed.

2.   The DEA has since taken over the whole hotel.

3.   Robert Gelbard finished his term in Bolivia in July 1991 and was replaced by Charles Bower.

4.   Interview with US official.

5.   'Guns, drugs and politics,' *Newsweek*, 28 July 1986.

6.   Ibid.

7. Ibid.

8. US House Committee on Foreign Affairs, *Operation Snowcap: past, present and future*, 23 May 1990.

9. Ibid.

10. M. Levine, *Deep Cover*, Delacorte Press, 1990.

11. US House Committee on Foreign Affairs, *Operation Snowcap: past, present and future*, 23 May 1990.

12. US Congressional Committee on Government Operations, *Stopping the flood of cocaine with Operation Snowcap: is it working?* 14 August 1990.

13. US House Committee on Foreign Affairs, *Operation Snowcap: past, present and future*, 23 May 1990.

14. Interview with Mike Levine published in *Extra*, July/August 1990.

15. 'DEA agents lead frustrating fight in Bolivian coca-growing region,' *Washington Post*, 16 January 1989.

16. 'US expands role in Peru's drug war,' *Washington Post*, 23 January 1989.

17. Ibid.

18. 'The drug busters,' *Newsweek*, 16 July 1990.

19. 'Special forces reportedly have joined Bolivian raids,' *Baltimore Sun*, 14 September 1989.

20 'The army's drug war,' *Army Times*, 2 October 1989.

21. Defense Policy Panel and Investigations Subcommittee, House Committee on Armed Services, *The Andean drug strategy and the role of the US military*, January 1990.

22. US Congressional Committee on Government Operations, *Stopping the flood of cocaine with Operation Snowcap: is it working?* 14 August 1990.

23. DOS Inspector General Report, March 1989.

24. 'The drug busters,' *Newsweek*, 16 July 1990.

Chapter 8

1. Information used as the basis of this chapter is from a senior US official who asked not to be named.

2. 'Blunt assessment of Bolivia ignored,' *Washington Post*, 1 March 1990.

3. The Bolivian economist Edmundo Morales estimates the value of cocaine to the Bolivian economy at $300 million, or 10-12 per cent of GNP. One US official puts it at $200-$600 million. Gonzálo Sánchez de Lozada, head of the MNR party, puts it at between $300 and $600 million.

Index